# HOW TO PREPARE FOR
# THE NEXT
# PANDEMIC

Behavioural Sciences Insights
for Practitioners and Policymakers

# HOW TO PREPARE FOR
# THE NEXT PANDEMIC

## Behavioural Sciences Insights for Practitioners and Policymakers

Edited by

### Majeed Khader
Home Team Behavioural Sciences Centre, Singapore
Nanyang Technological University, Singapore

### Denise Dillon
James Cook University, Singapore

### Xingyu Ken Chen
Home Team Behavioural Sciences Centre, Singapore

### Loo Seng Neo
Home Team Behavioural Sciences Centre, Singapore

### Jeffery Chin
Home Team Behavioural Sciences Centre, Singapore

**World Scientific**

NEW JERSEY · LONDON · SINGAPORE · BEIJING · SHANGHAI · HONG KONG · TAIPEI · CHENNAI · TOKYO

*Published by*

World Scientific Publishing Co. Pte. Ltd.

5 Toh Tuck Link, Singapore 596224

*USA office:* 27 Warren Street, Suite 401-402, Hackensack, NJ 07601

*UK office:* 57 Shelton Street, Covent Garden, London WC2H 9HE

**Library of Congress Cataloging-in-Publication Data**

Names: Khader, Majeed, 1966–  editor.

Title: How to prepare for the next pandemic : behavioural sciences insights for practitioners and
   policymakers / edited by Majeed Khader, Home Team Behavioural Sciences Centre and
   Nanyang Technological University, Singapore, Denise Dillon, James Cook University,
   Singapore, Xingyu Ken Chen, Loo Seng Neo, Jeffery Chin, Home Team Behavioural
   Sciences Centre, Singapore.

Description: New Jersey : World Scientific, [2021] | Includes bibliographical references.

Identifiers: LCCN 2020045919 | ISBN 9789811230042 (hardcover) |
   ISBN 9789811230059 (ebook) | ISBN 9789811230066 (ebook other)

Subjects: LCSH: COVID-19 (Disease) | COVID-19 (Disease)--Psychological aspects. |
   COVID-19 (Disease)--Social aspects. | COVID-19 (Disease)--Political aspects. |
   COVID-19 (Disease)--Economic aspects. | Preparedness.

Classification: LCC RA644.C67 H69 2021 | DDC 614.5/92414--dc23

LC record available at https://lccn.loc.gov/2020045919

**British Library Cataloguing-in-Publication Data**

A catalogue record for this book is available from the British Library.

For any available supplementary material, please visit
https://www.worldscientific.com/worldscibooks/10.1142/12094#t=suppl

Desk Editors: Balamurugan Rajendran/Karimah Samsudin

Typeset by Stallion Press
Email: enquiries@stallionpress.com

# About the Editors

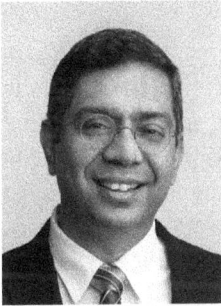

**Majeed Khader** is the Director of the Home Team Behavioural Sciences Centre under the Ministry of Home Affairs (MHA), Singapore. Dr Majeed is also the Chief Psychologist of the MHA. A trained hostage negotiator, his previous operational duties include being the Deputy Commander of the Crisis Negotiation Unit and a trainer with the negotiation unit. He teaches criminal psychology as an Assistant Professor (Adjunct) at the School of Social Sciences at Nanyang Technology University (NTU), Singapore. For the past 26 years, Majeed has overseen the development of psychological services in the areas of stress, resilience, employee selection, deception psychology, leadership, crisis negotiations, crime profiling, and crisis psychology. For his work, he was awarded the National Day Public Administration Award (Bronze) in 2006 by the President of Singapore, and once again the Public Administration Award Silver in 2014. A pioneer forensic psychologist, Majeed holds a Master's degree (with Distinction) in Forensic Psychology from the University of Leicester (United Kingdom), and a PhD in Psychology (specialising in personality and crisis leadership) from the University of Aberdeen, Scotland. Majeed has been invited as a speaker to organisations in Indonesia, Malaysia, Japan, Canada, Hong Kong, United Kingdom, and the United States to share on crime psychology, terrorism, and leadership. He has also presented at the FBI, NCIS, and the RCMP. He has been the Chairman of the Asian Conference of Criminal and Operations Psychology thrice. He is the Asian Director of the United States-based Society of Police and Criminal Psychology, and a member of the Asia Pacific Association of Threat Assessment Professionals. He is a Registered Psychologist with the Singapore Psychological Society (SPS), and a member of the British, and American Psychological Societies. He has contributed to several book chapters and published widely in peer-reviewed journal such as *Journal of Research in Personality, Journal of Occupational Health Psychology, Psychology & Health, Cognition and Emotion, International Journal of Psychophysiology, Personality and Individual Differences, International Journal of Police Science & Management, Journal of Police and Criminal Psychology*, and *Security Journal*.

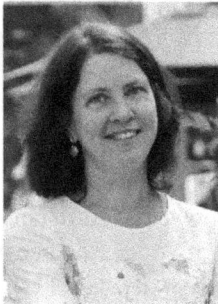

**Denise Dillon** is an academic living and working in Singapore, at James Cook University. In 2020, she led a research team on national and international survey-based research to study the psychosocial effects of COVID-19. An environmental psychologist by training, Dr Dillon is also a literary critic by heart, and she publishes in the field of ecocriticism as well as in her specific areas of research interest, in environmental psychology and biophilia. Dr Dillon is a member of the Singapore Psychological Society (SPS) Council, and currently holds the position of Research Chair.

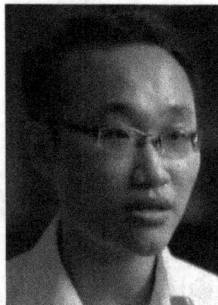

**Xingyu Ken Chen** is a Senior Behavioural Sciences Research Analyst at the Home Team Behavioural Sciences Centre, Ministry of Home Affairs (MHA), Singapore. Some of his other writings include psychological vulnerabilities to fake news in the aftermath of a terror attack in *Learning from Violent Extremist Attacks: Behavioural Sciences Insights for Practitioners and Policymakers* (2018), the intersection of crime and fake news in *Encyclopaedia of Criminal Activities and the Deep Web*. His current research interests include online misinformation,

information operations, strategic communications, and natural language processing.

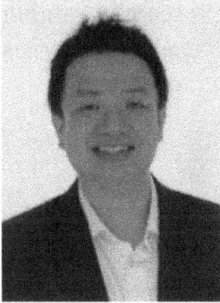

**Loo Seng Neo** is a Principal Behavioural Sciences Research Analyst with the Home Team Behavioural Sciences Centre at the Ministry of Home Affairs (MHA), Singapore. For the past 13 years, Loo Seng has been leading a team of research analysts and interns to research on emergent trends on terrorism, resilience, misinformation, and intergroup conflict, and distilling useful insights for the ministry through research reports and training for law enforcement officers. He has also trained grassroots leaders and the general public about the threat of terrorism and how to prepare for the "day after" terror. Based on his research, Loo Seng has presented at many international conferences and published many peer-reviewed journals and book chapters. He has also co-edited several books. He is currently pursuing his PhD in psychology at the Nanyang Technological University (NTU), Singapore, where he attempts to identify person-centric, psychosocial, and protective factors that can identify markers of radicalisation in social media posts. In his spare time, he mentors psychology undergraduates from the local universities.

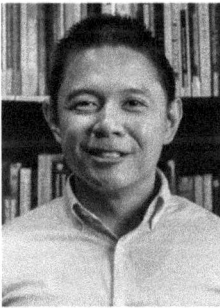

**Jeffery Chin** has been a staff Psychologist with the Home Team Behavioural Sciences Centre (HTBSC) since 2006. Incepted in 2006, the HTBSC is an applied behavioural sciences research, training and operational support unit in the Ministry of Home Affairs (MHA), Singapore. One of the Centre's key remit is to translate knowledge from the field of psychology and the behavioural sciences into operational knowledge that law enforcement, safety, security, and correctional agencies under the auspices of MHA may utilise or incorporate into their policies, operations, and practice. As one of the pioneers at the HTBSC, Jeffery played an important role in setting up the unit in its initial years, and oversaw its development from a programme (the Behavioural Sciences Programme) in 2006 to a full-fledged psychological research and training centre (the Home Team Behavioural

Sciences Centre) presently. He has been involved in roles and projects across several domains that supported the operations and development of Singapore law enforcement and security officers over the years. The roles and projects include crime and investigation support research, training and consultation, crisis intervention and resilience management, crisis negotiation operations, and leadership development and assessment.

# About the Contributors

**Whistine Chai** is a Lead Psychologist with the Crime, Investigation and Forensic Psychology Branch of the Home Team Behavioural Sciences Centre. Currently leading the branch as Assistant Director, she fronts projects relating to forensic and investigative psychology, and seeks to apply psychological and behavioural sciences principles in understanding and enhancing investigative support tools and initiatives for the Ministry. Other key areas of her work include applied research in risk assessment, threat assessment, cybercrimes and scams. A graduate of the National University of Singapore, she also holds a master's degree (with Distinction) in Clinical Forensic Psychology from the Institute of Psychiatry, Psychology & Neuroscience, King's College London, where, she won two awards—the John Gunn Prize for Highest Overall Mark in the cohort, and the Sheilagh Hodgins Prize for Highest Dissertation Mark in the programme.

**Cherie Chan** is the current President of the Singapore Psychological Society (SPS) and a registered Clinical Psychologist and Supervisor with the Singapore Register of Psychologists (SRP). During the COVID-19 pandemic, Cherie has worked to push for the recognition of psychological services to be an essential service in Singapore and has provided pro-bono services, supervised on the National Care Hotline, and provided specialised webinars and talks for the public to gain awareness of the importance of mental health and role of psychologists through these unprecedented times. In the last decade, Cherie has worked in the public sector, teaches undergraduate and masters students, and currently provides therapy for adults and adolescents in a private clinic setting.

**Damien D. Cheong** is a Research Fellow and Acting Head of the National Security Studies Programme (NSSP), S. Rajaratnam School of International Studies (RSIS), Nanyang Technological University (NTU), Singapore. Prior to this, he was Research Fellow and Coordinator of the Homeland Defence Programme at the Centre of Excellence for National Security (CENS) at RSIS from 2011–2017. He has researched and written on various topics related to homeland security, strategic communication and political violence. His current research focuses on small state security.

**Oindrila Dutta** is a Doctoral Researcher in Psychology at Nanyang Technological University (NTU), Singapore. She has completed her Masters in Counselling and Guidance and is also a Certified Thanatologist of the Association for Death Education and Counseling (ADEC). She serves as the committee chair for the ADEC Student and New Professionals Committee's Social Media & Outreach Division. Oindrila is passionate about employing culturally sensitive approaches to improve quality of life and holistic well-being for patients and their families who are facing end-of-life and mortality. Her research contributions include proposing the Trauma to Transformation model of Asian parental bereavement and piloting the novel Narrative e-Writing Intervention (NeW-I) for advancing paediatric palliative care and grief support services in Singapore. Her past experiences include psychotherapy in a University Counselling Center to help young adults, particularly international students, build resilience and cope with typical life challenges. In recognition of her work, Oindrila has received numerous commendations including the Best Cross-Cultural Student Paper Award by ADEC (2019) and the Dean's Commendation for Research by the National Institute of Education, Singapore (2017).

**Paul Englert** is a Lecturer at the Department of Psychology, Nanyang Technological University (NTU), Singapore. Born and educated in New Zealand, Paul has over two decades of experience in the field of industrial and organisational (I/O) psychology. He is a published academic writer with 20 articles and book chapters currently in publication. His speciality is psychometrics; and he has published in areas as diverse as cognitive ability, personality, and cultural differences in psychometric tests. Paul is very proud to be part of a business that continues to forge new ground both in New Zealand and across the world by sticking to its core values of applied research and practical application of I/O Psychology solutions. Professionally, Paul is known as a Pracademic; as he is both a practitioner and an academic, and in working with clients, he brings an eclectic mix of business experience, academic backing, and innovative problem solving. Paul heads programmes in psychometrics, personality and individual differences, the psychology of leadership, the psychology of conflict and resolution, and the psychology of personnel selection. He has also developed a practicum course for the training of I/O psychologists in Singapore.

**Pamela Goh** is a Behavioural Sciences Research Analyst with the Home Team Behavioural Sciences Centre (HTBSC), Ministry of Home Affairs (MHA), Singapore. Her research experience and repertoire in the organisation includes building national resilience in relation to nation-wide crises, as well as understanding the phenomenon of social movements. Some of her past work included crowd behaviours during crises, building social cohesion, and crisis communications. Additionally, she has delved into the area of whole-of-society engagement in response to crises, and has organised two roundtables involving academics, governmental officials, non-governmental organisations, and other law-enforcement agencies, to discuss community responses to terror attacks. Pamela is currently pursuing her PhD at the Nanyang Technological University (NTU), with an avid interest in community resilience and cohesion in times of crises. As part of her dissertation, she is looking at understanding whether and why people would act for themselves or for others during times of threatened survival, such as a terror attack.

**Andy Hau Yan Ho** is Associate Professor of Psychology and Medicine at Nanyang Technological University (NTU), Singapore. He serves as Board Director of the Association for Death Education and Counselling (ADEC) and the International Work Group on Death Dying and Bereavement (IWGDDB). Andy's expertise lies in psychosocial gerontology, palliative and bereavement care, holistic interventions, and community empowerment. He is the founder of numerous innovative and acclaimed psycho-socio-spiritual interventions that promote capacity building, including Mindful-Compassion Art-based Therapy (MCAT) for burnout prevention and resilience building among caregivers; Family Dignity Intervention (FDI) for advancing holistic end-of-life care; Narrative e-Writing Intervention (NeW-I) for enhancing paediatric palliative care; and Aspiration and Resilience Through Intergenerational Storytelling and Art-based Narratives (ARTISAN) for citizen empowerment. Andy has authored over 100 top-tier journal articles, books, chapters, and research reports; and presented in over 180 keynote, plenary, and competitive conference presentations. He is the first Asian Recipient of the eminent "ADEC Academic Educator Award" in 2018, while capturing the prestigious "Nanyang Education Award" in 2019, and conferred the "Distinguished Alumni Award" from the University of Hong Kong in 2020. Andy's social and scholarly contributions are recognised with distinction by professional bodies around the world.

**Minzheng Hou** is a Doctoral Candidate in Social Psychology at the National University of Singapore (NUS) and a recipient of the President's Graduate Fellowship. His core research area resides in motivation and decision-making. A member of the Situated Goal Pursuit Lab, he is also actively involved in research projects aimed at enhancing intergroup relations based on motivation science. Prior to pursuing his PhD, Minzheng was at the Institute of Policy Studies (IPS), Lee Kuan Yew School of Public Policy (LKYSPP), where he spearheaded national level surveys on social resilience. Minzheng also served as a Naval Officer in the Republic of Singapore Navy for more than seven years where he was actively deployed for frontline operations and intimately involved in operational policy development. Minzheng obtained his Bachelor's degree (highest honours) in Psychology and Economics from the University of Michigan, Ann Arbor. During his time at Michigan, he received the prestigious Goldstein Prize (Marshall Sahlins Social Science Award) as a recognition of his academic and research achievements.

**Ghee Kian Koh** is a Singaporean student currently completing his Honours for the Bachelor of Psychological Science, at James Cook University. As a fourth-year psychology undergraduate, he has been trained in the analysis and application of social psychology theories. Mr. Koh is an avid supporter of environmental sustainability and green transition, keenly exploring psychology's role in crises arising from climate change, and COVID-19 now. Mr. Koh aspires to pursue a career as an environmental or conservation psychologist.

**Jonathan Han Loong Kuek** is a Doctoral Candidate at the University of Sydney, specialising in recovery approaches to the management and understanding of mental health conditions. He is a published author and serves as a journal reviewer for other peer reviewed journals. Jonathan has been involved in international conferences where his oral presentations and posters have been selected for presentation. He is an active mental health advocate who has been volunteering with the Institute of Mental Health (IMH) for the past six years where he founded a youth volunteering group. Jonathan is a mentor to undergraduate psychology students under the SGP Psych Stuff mentorship programme which he is currently in charge of. He is an active member of the Singapore Psychological Society (SPS) as part of the public education team and frequently gives talks about careers and topics in psychology. Jonathan also has extensive experience working within the social service sector and has worked alongside many agencies in the mental health sector. He believes strongly in the need for greater involvement by people experiencing mental health conditions when services and policies are planned for, and constantly advocates for their right to do so.

**Dymples Leong** is a Senior Analyst with the Centre of Excellence for National Security (CENS) at the S. Rajaratnam School of International Studies (RSIS), Nanyang Technological University (NTU), Singapore. Her research focuses on behavioural insights and policymaking, social media, and strategic communications. Her commentaries have been published in The Straits Times, The Diplomat, Channel NewsAsia, The Interpreter, East Asia Forum and the Asian Journal of Pacific Affairs. Dymples holds a Bachelor of Business majoring in Marketing and Management from the University of Newcastle, Australia.

**Jose Ma. Luis Montesclaros**, MPP is Associate Research Fellow with the Centre of Non-Traditional Security Studies (NTS Centre), S. Rajaratnam School of International Studies (RSIS), Nanyang Technological University (NTU), Singapore. He conducts policy analysis with dynamic models of food security, economics, agriculture, and climate change in ASEAN, and has provided inputs to Singapore's Inter-Ministry Committee on Food Security (IMCFS). He is also First

Inventor of the UrbanAgInvest tool (© NTU) tool, developed to facilitate state investments into high-tech farming sectors, together with Professor Paul Teng (Co-Inventor). Prior to joining RSIS, he was consultant to the World Bank's Trade and Competitiveness Global Practice Group in Singapore, and to the Chief Economist Office for East Asia and the Pacific (headquartered in Washington D.C.), and co-author of the Bank's ASEAN-Commissioned report, "Bridging the Development Gap: ASEAN Equitable Development Monitor Report 2014". He holds a Master's Degree in Public Policy from the Lee Kuan Yew School of Public Policy (LKYSPP), National University of Singapore (NUS) (ASEAN Scholar), where he was one of the LKYSPP's two "Leaders of Tomorrow" representatives at the 44th St. Gallen Wings of Leadership Awards at the University of St. Gallen, Switzerland. He also holds a BS Economics Degree from the University of the Philippines, Diliman.

**Stephanie Neubronner** is a Research Fellow in the National Security Studies Programme at the S. Rajaratnam School of International Studies (RSIS), Nanyang Technological University (NTU), Singapore. Her research interests include sociocultural identity, governance and social relations, and the influence of new media. Stephanie obtained first class honours in Anthropology and Sociology from the University of Western Australia (UWA). She was subsequently awarded UWA's Postgraduate Award Scholarship and completed her PhD in Anthropology, Sociology and Geography. Prior to joining RSIS, Stephanie was a researcher at the Institute of Policy Studies (IPS), Lee Kuan Yew School of Public Policy (LKYSPP), National University of Singapore (NUS).

**Shannon Ng** is a Behavioural Sciences Research Analyst with the Home Team Behavioural Sciences Centre (HTBSC) at the Ministry of Home Affairs (MHA), Singapore. Shannon graduated from the Nanyang Technological University with a Bachelor of Arts in English with Honours (Distinction) and a minor in Psychology. Her current field of research covers cyber-related crimes and violent crimes—in their emergence, deviancy and prevention/ interception. Some of her work includes research on emerging cybercrime trends like image-based sexual abuse and cyber scams. Her interests lie in criminal profiling and youth offending, and how power dynamics of race, age, gender, social class etc. contributes to crime and its solutioning.

**Paul Victor Patinadan** is a Doctoral Researcher at the School of Social Science, Nanyang Technological University (NTU), funded by the Ministry of Education (MOE), Singapore. He is also a certified Thanatologist of the Association for Death Education and Counselling (ADEC). As a mixed-methods researcher, Paul specialises in holistic palliative and end-of-life care, life and death education, and psychosocial interventions and therapies. His current work focuses on a novel Family Dignity Intervention (FDI) directed at providing patients and their families within the palliative care health ecosystem of Singapore nuanced psycho-socio-spiritual support. He has also worked on several projects with a focus on health psychology, including health technology-based behaviours of the chronically ill and a national evaluation of Singapore's Advance Care Planning programme. To date, he has participated in several international and local conferences, and has been awarded with a number of honours, including the prestigious Santander Mobility Grant (2019) and first place for his presentation during the 3 Minute Thesis competition at his alma mater (2014). As reflected in his continuing research pursuits, Paul holds special interest in the mediums of food, humour and technology as dignity-enhancing and legacy-building tools for individuals taking their final steps in life's journey.

**Nur Aisyah Abdul Rahman** is currently a Behavioural Sciences Research Analyst at the Home Team Behavioural Sciences Centre (HTBSC). She has an undergraduate degree in Psychology. Aisyah's areas of research involve social cohesion issues in light of violent extremism (e.g., prejudice, Islamophobia), microaggressions, and right-wing extremism. She is part of a team that regularly conducts seminars and trainings for police officers, religious and community leaders. She enjoys learning more about violent extremism and related social phenomenon. She has also published and contributed to several reports, journal articles, and book chapters on topics related to violent extremism and social cohesion, as well as presenting her research findings at various conferences and seminars.

**Jonathan E. Ramsay** is a Senior Lecturer of Psychology and the Academic Head for the School of Social and Health Sciences at James Cook University, Singapore. Originally from the United Kingdom,

Dr. Ramsay has spent the last 11 years living and working in Singapore. He received a PhD in Psychology from Nanyang Technological University (NTU) in 2014, and a BA in psychology and physiology from the University of Oxford in 2005. His research interests span areas of personality and social psychology, with a particular emphasis on the psychology of religion and the relationships between personality, attitudes, and well-being. His current research projects examine the way religious individuals explain daily events, as well as individual differences in the relationship between subjective authenticity and well-being. Dr. Ramsay has published in many international peer-reviewed journals, such as Nature Human Behaviour, the Journal of Personality, and Political Psychology. He is an editorial board member for the Asian Journal of Social Psychology and the International Journal for the Psychology of Religion, and regularly reviews for journals such as Motivation and Emotion and the Journal of Pacific Rim Psychology. He is also the recipient of several internal and external research grants.

**Vivian Seah** is a Psychologist with the Crime, Investigation, and Forensic Psychology (CIFP) Branch of the Home Team Behavioural Sciences Centre (HTBSC). Key areas of her work at HTBSC include crime and behavioural analysis, and behavioural sciences research on scams, drugs and organised crime. Her research interests also include the detection of deception and investigative interviewing. She organises and conducts trainings for Home Team officers in the area of crime and behavioural analysis. Through her work in HTBSC, she engages the community to build interest in the area of investigative and forensic psychology by being part of the organising committee of the annual Criminal Behavioural Analysis Competition (CBAC) and the Asian Conference of Criminal and Operations Psychology (ACCOP) 2019. She is a trained volunteer Victim Care Officer (VCO) with the Singapore Police Force, where she provides psychological support to victims of crimes. She is also a psychologist with the Singapore Police Force Crisis Negotiation Unit, where she is involved in crisis negotiation operations by giving psychological inputs during negotiations.

**Geraldine Tan-Ho** is Senior Counsellor and Research Associate of Psychology at Nanyang Technological University, Singapore. She is a

Certified Thanatologist of the Association for Death Education and Counseling (ADEC), and serves as Co-Chair of the Community Engagement and Communication Committee of the Singapore Hospice Council (SHC). A passionate advocate for quality of life and quality of death, Geraldine has rich experience in community action and social change, as she was previously a Medical Social Worker and Counsellor for low-income families, sick elderly, terminally ill children and caregivers. As a Counsellor in Singapore's biggest paediatric palliative home care team, she restructured and developed national standards of excellence in bereavement care for caregivers and families of children and young adults who died from various chronic life-limiting conditions. Currently, Geraldine focuses her efforts on pioneering a novel Family Dignity Intervention (FDI) for older terminally ill patients and their families, as well as developing an innovative Narrative e-Writing Intervention (NeW-I) for advancing holistic paediatric palliative care and parental bereavement support services, with the ultimate goal to address the culture-specific psycho-socio-spiritual needs of Asian populations facing loss and mortality.

**Jessie Janny Thenarianto** is a Behavioural Sciences Research Analyst at the Home Team Behavioural Sciences Centre (HTBSC). She graduated summa cum laude from Universitas Ciputra, Indonesia, with a bachelor's degree in Psychology. Her current research interests include crisis, resilience, human behaviour in cyberspace, and crime. Some of her published works include the social media response after the 2016 and 2017 Jakarta bombings in Learning from Violent Extremist Attacks: Behavioural Sciences Insights for Practitioners and Policymakers (2018) and political symbolism on social media during elections in Psikologi dan Integrasi Bangsa: Seri Sumbangan Pemikiran Psikologi untuk Bangsa 4 (2020).

**Adrian Toh** is a Registered Clinical Psychologist who works closely with individuals with health and mental health issues in the last decade. He serves in the Singapore Psychological Society (SPS) as the Chairperson for Singapore Register of Psychologists (SRP). During the COVID-19 pandemic, Adrian was privileged to walk alongside with patients affected by the disease, and to lead teams in providing psychological care to frontline healthcare workers. During the same period, he was also involved in manning the National Care Hotline, initiating pro-bono counselling services and writing articles regarding coping with the pandemic. Adrian's personal experience with pandemics include having children born during the Zika outbreak and COVID-19.

**John Yu** is a Psychologist with the Crime, Investigation, and Forensic Psychology branch of the Home Team Behavioural Sciences Centre. John graduated from the National University of Singapore with a Bachelor of Social Sciences (Honours) in Psychology. His research interest lies in emerging criminal and deviant behaviours of concern. He also conducts training for law enforcement officers in criminal and forensic psychology. John is a co-organiser of the Criminal Behavioural Analysis Competition in Singapore, an annual nationwide competition that introduces tertiary students and undergraduates to criminal profiling and investigative techniques, psychological first aid, and crisis negotiation skills.

# Acknowledgements

It has been a privilege for us to work on this emerging but important topic on responding to the COVID-19 health crisis. The completion of this book would not be possible without the support of everyone who has contributed in one way or another. This book is a testament to the strong support we have received from our research partners and colleagues working in the field of psychology. Therefore, we would like to acknowledge everyone who has played a critical role in the completion of this book.

It has been a remarkable journey for us, and we would like to first express our most heartfelt gratitude towards our authors for their contributions to this book. A huge thanks to all our authors for your expertise, open-handedness, passion, and patience. It has been a great pleasure working with you, and we are grateful for your faith in this project. We would also like to thank World Scientific Publishing, the publisher of this book, and in particular, Ms. Karimah Samsudin, the editor who has supported us tirelessly throughout this book project.

Next, we would wish to acknowledge those who have contributed to the various stages of the production process. A number of the Home Team Behavioural Sciences Centre (HTBSC) colleagues have graciously offered their time, insights, and administrative support to this project. We want to acknowledge Mr. Hou Minzheng and Ms. Pamela Goh for their valuable assistance and reviews that have greatly improved the coherence and readability of the book. Ms. Halitha Banu, Ms. Lee Jing Yi, and Ms. Samantha Lim have also been a huge support in providing valuable inputs on the formatting and proof-reading issues during the final edit of the book. We would also like to thank Mr. Chan Chunmu for his kind administrative support. Last but not least, our sincere appreciation to all our colleagues at HTBSC for their personal, professional, and moral support towards this project.

In addition, we wish to highlight that this project is not an official government endeavour, and thus the views expressed here represent the views of the authors and editors only. The chapters of this book do not represent the official views of the Government of Singapore in any way. Notwithstanding that, we are grateful for our management's support and encouragement towards our work and research. We are also thankful for the support from Ms. Chua Lee Hoong, Dr. Ng Yih Yng, our valued-partners from MHA (Joint Training Centre [JTC], Heritage Development Unit [HDU]), the National Security Studies Programme (NSSP), the Centre of Excellence for National Security (CENS), James Cook University (JCU), and the Singapore Psychological Society (SPS). At Nanyang Technological University (NTU), our thanks go to Associate Professor Joyce Pang, Associate Professor Ringo Ho, and Associate Professor Kumar Ramakrishna for their support and guidance.

Finally, we would like to take this opportunity to thank the members of our families. Majeed is deeply thankful to Leong Tscheng Yee, Tasneem, and Raouf, and his mum Hawa, for their unconditional love and support. Denise is eternally thankful to her parents, who are gone but never forgotten. Ken is grateful to his parents, Hua Soon and Siew Nuan, for their love and support. Jeffery is grateful to his wife, Mol, for her love, understanding, and unwavering support. Loo Seng is deeply indebted to his wife, Onpapha, and his three children, Xi Zhen, An Qi, and An Ping, for their love and support. We truly appreciate their invaluable support and love.

To our readers, thank you for taking the time to read this book. We hope you find our humble project a pleasure to read!

# Contents

# Introduction

# How to Prepare for the Next Pandemic: Behavioural Sciences Insights for Practitioners and Policymakers

Xingyu Ken Chen, Loo Seng Neo, and Jeffery Chin

## The Wicked Problem of COVID-19

The COVID-19 outbreak has highlighted how various spheres of life, such as public health, economics, employment, community, and even mental health, are closely intertwined. With tens of millions infected and thousands dying from the virus worldwide, COVID-19 has not only put pressure on the healthcare systems around the world, it has also affected many aspects of contemporary life. These include the contraction of the global economy, the disruption of communal harmony, negative impact on the psychological well-being of members of the public, and difficulties in keeping the public updated of the evolving pandemic situation.

Rittel and Webber (1973) coined the term "wicked problem" to refer to issues that are difficult to solve, not because the problem is inherently difficult, but because such issues do not offer themselves up to solutions. A wicked problem is complex and its causes may be multifaceted and nebulous. Grappling with its effects would therefore demand the input of multiple disciplines as no one perspective is sufficient to enhance our understanding and ability to deal with it. In this sense, the COVID-19 pandemic can be labelled as a wicked problem.

There are a few features of the pandemic which makes it such a problem. Firstly, lessons drawn from past experience in mitigating the spread of pandemics, such as the Severe Acute Respiratory Syndrome (SARS), are often limited in effectiveness due to the role of other factors in exacerbating the current COVID-19 situation. With no specific treatment currently available and the estimates for a viable vaccine being at least 12 to 18 months away (Ghosh & Tan, 2020), as of the time of the writing of this book, social distancing will continue to play a dominant role in curbing the spread of infection, while fundamentally affecting the economic, putting a strain on the healthcare systems, and causing communal tensions within the society. These developments make it a daunting task for authorities to effectively respond to the pandemic.

The second being that solutions for wicked problems are seldom true or false, but rather they reflect trade-offs between better or worse solutions. This can be seen in the multitude of second-order effects that followed after countries implemented movement restriction measures to contain the pandemic, which profoundly transformed the way society was organised. It has significantly disrupted the operations of many businesses and organisations. Many companies have been forced to embrace telecommuting as the default mode of work as part of their business continuity plans. Furthermore, organisations have downsized their businesses to cope with changes in demands, leading many to lose their jobs (Iacurci, 2020). In the same vein, with around one-third of the world's population experiencing movement restriction measures, millions of households are likely to experience increased stress, anxiety, anger, irritability, emotional exhaustion, depression, and post-traumatic stress (Hoof, 2020). It is clear that the wicked problem posed by the COVID-19 pandemic cannot be understood in isolation, and solutions cannot be created in institutional silos.

In Singapore, a massive effort was mounted by the government to mitigate the effects of COVID-19. Among the many public health-related interventions, such as the circuit breaker measure to stem the rising rates of community transmissions in April and the ramping up of testing capacity (Lai, 2020), various policies and measures were made to address the systemic effects brought about by the pandemic. For instance, in the space of a few months, the Singapore government passed four stimulus bills, spending nearly S$100 billion to support the economy and workers (Lee, 2020). These stimulus bills were funded by drawing on national reserves, an action that only occurred once in Singapore's entire history during the 2007–2008 Global Financial Crisis, highlighting the economic severity of the current situation.

Members of the public, as well as private organisations, have also been involved in the fight against COVID-19. During the first five months of the pandemic, the public has stepped up to help those in need. In fact, they have donated S$90 million to the Community Chest and Giving.sg. This amount is equal to the total amount of donations that those organisations received in the entire 2019 (Goh, 2020). The SGUnited movement was also established to rally Singaporeans. This initiative allowed Singaporeans to come together to help one another in the face of the health crisis—e.g., volunteering in various organic campaigns. People were also collectively involved in showing appreciation for the frontliners, by clapping their hands and singing songs from the windows of their homes during the circuit breaker period ("Sing along to Home", 2020).

However, the fight against COVID-19 is far from over. Other challenges loom ahead as the pandemic persists. The contraction of the global economy means that many businesses are likely to struggle and even stop their operations, with retrenchment and increasing unemployment rates being unavoidable realities for many countries, including Singapore. This can create psychological stress among those who are affected by these new developments. In other words, there is an urgent need to increase our understanding of this wicked problem of COVID-19, and identify solutions informed by a multidisciplinary approach to mitigate the negative consequences on various fronts such as the economic, healthcare systems, community harmony, and individual's well-being.

## The Need for a Behavioural Sciences Approach

In view of this wicked problem, a pragmatic and collaborative effort is therefore required to conceive answers to respond and mitigate the impact of COVID-19, and to prepare for the next pandemic. Various experts have opined that social and behavioural sciences have been overlooked by many in their efforts to contain COVID-19 (Bais, 2020; Balkhi *et al.*, 2020). For instance, in a recent publication in Nature Human Behaviour, Bavel and colleagues (2020) underscored the importance of adopting a behavioural sciences approach:

> Insights from the past century of work on related issues in the social and behavioural sciences that may help public health officials mitigate the impact of the current pandemic. Specifically, we discussed research on

threat perception, social context, science communication, aligning individual and collective interests, leadership, and stress and coping ... Urgent action is needed to mitigate the potentially devastating effects of COVID-19, action that can be supported by the behavioural and social sciences. (p. 467)

As such, this book, titled *How to Prepare for the Next Pandemic: Behavioural Sciences Insights for Practitioners and Policymakers*, attempts to contribute to the existing literature by offering a behavioural sciences approach to enhance our response to the threat of pandemics, with knowledge drawn from diverse fields—e.g., psychology, sociology, history, political science, technology, and communications. This would then help to identify scientifically defensible interventions and approaches for both the practitioners and policymakers. Seventeen chapters will be introduced in this book. These chapters attempt to shed light on how practitioners, policymakers, academics, and members of the public can understand issues and strategies to (1) foster societal resilience, (2) build their psychological well-being, (3) use information found in the digital sphere, and (4) enhance the functioning of their organisations. Every single chapter is premised on the view that insights from these research areas have something to contribute to the overall effort of preparing for the next pandemic.

There are three ways in which this book adds value to the existing literature. Firstly, this book recognises the complexity undermining the wicked problem of pandemics, and aims to provide a multidisciplinary approach to the issue at hand. Of particular value is the confluence of perspectives from psychologists, political scientists, sociologists, and communications experts. This will provide readers with greater confidence on the steps needed to understand and mitigate this problem. It also complements the valuable findings from similar scholarship, such as the book by Professor David Chan titled *Combating a Crisis: The Psychology of Singapore's Response to COVID-19*. Secondly, this book encapsulates an endeavour to solicit and harness the insights of practitioners, policymakers, and subject matter experts in their field of research. The contributors share their perspectives and wealth of experiences that could enrich and act as a critical and timely resource to inform strategies to combat COVID-19 and future pandemics. Lastly, this book aims to provide insights from a Singaporean perspective such that the information presented will be relevant to local practitioners, policymakers, academics, and members of the public. To this end, the editors (from the Home Team Behavioural Sciences Centre, Ministry of Home Affairs, together with James Cook University [Singapore]) have invited local partners to contribute chapters to the topic of preparing for pandemics, where much of the research has originated from the Western perspective.

These three points underscore the *raison d'être* behind this book, and to ensure that the content is accessible to the targeted audience of practitioners, policymakers, and members of the public, the chapters are written in a short and succinct manner. More importantly, the editors seek to convey a spirit of openness, wherein the contributors are strongly encouraged to share any useful insights that have not yet been heard of or which runs contrary to prevailing conventional views. Instead of echoing conventional views, this approach acknowledges the rich and varied range of disparate questions and issues associated with mitigating the threat of pandemics, and serves as a starting point for readers to reflect and envision new areas of research and/or strategies to protect themselves and their loved ones.

## Organisation of the Book

The chapters have been organised broadly into the following sections:

- Section 1: Societal Resilience Related Issues (Chapters 1 to 4)
- Section 2: Psychological Well-Being Related Issues (Chapters 5 to 8)
- Section 3: Digital Communication Related Issues (Chapters 9 to 12)
- Section 4: Organisational Related Issues (Chapters 13 to 16)
- Section 5: Future Directions (Chapter 17).

### *Societal Resilience Related Issues*

In the first four chapters, attention is directed towards issues and strategies surrounding efforts to foster societal resilience in times of a pandemic. Denise Dillon and Ghee Kian Koh's opening chapter on "A Journal of the COVID Year: What Can We Learn from Previous Pandemics?" (Chapter 1) examines the current COVID-19 situation based on three types of psychosocial reactions to epidemics, and how these reactions were observed in past pandemics such as SARS and

MERS. They then shed light on the occurrence of these psychosocial reactions in COVID-19, and provide insights on how authorities should react to them. Jose Montesclaros in his chapter "What are the Economic Impacts of a Pandemic?" (Chapter 2) explains the economic impacts of today's lockdown policies by discussing how economic disruptions brought upon by COVID-19 can spiral into economic crises, and the logic behind the interventions taken by governments to support businesses and the healthcare sector. Next, in the chapter "Enhancing Collective Community Resilience Throughout a Pandemic: Insights from Singapore" (Chapter 3), Pamela Goh discusses four strategies that individuals and community leaders can do to help in the containment of the health crisis. She opines that the adoption of these strategies could help to enhance community resilience and pave the way for the recovery process. Finally, Nur Aisyah in her chapter "Mitigating the Social Pandemic of Xenophobia During COVID-19" (Chapter 4) looks at the rise of virus-related prejudice and acts of discrimination using insights from the Integrated Threat Theory. In particular, she shares three strategies that could help authorities to alleviate the expression of prejudice and discrimination within our society.

### Psychological Well-Being Related Issues

In recent months, concerns about people's mental well-being are regularly discussed over many platforms. Bearing this in mind, Cherie Chan and Adrian Toh, in their chapter "How to Cope with Mental Health Issues During a Pandemic" (Chapter 5), focus on ways that individuals could do to cope with mental health issues during a pandemic, based on lessons learnt in this and past pandemics. They highlight practical steps to keep things in perspective, build personal resilience, improve coping styles, and care for vulnerable groups such as children. In the chapter "How to Support People with Mental Health Conditions During a Pandemic" (Chapter 6), Jonathan Kuek seeks to answer the question of how to support people experiencing mental health conditions, and explores the crucial role that mental health experts play in reducing the negative impact of a pandemic. Next, Jonathan Ramsay in his chapter "Coping with COVID-19: The Role of Religion in Times of Crisis" (Chapter 7) examines the intricacies associated with religious coping. In it, he applies important findings in the religious and spiritual coping literature to the local, regional, and global fight against COVID-19. Finally, Andy Ho,

Oindrila Dutta, Paul Victor Patinadan, and Geraldine Tan-Ho, in their chapter "Supporting and Coping with Bereavement During and Post-Pandemic" (Chapter 8), articulate the pain of disenfranchised grief arising from the implementation of social distancing measures, and outline how collective mourning and meaning reconstruction could aid in supporting and empowering bereavement recovery in a post-pandemic world.

## *Digital Communication Related Issues*

The central question underpinning the third section of the book revolves around the digital sphere, which plays an important role in helping individuals receive and comprehend information about COVID-19. In the chapter "The Role of Social Media During a Pandemic" (Chapter 9), Dymples Leong explores the nature of social media as a dynamic tool that provides valuable resource to people, as well as amplifies the propensity for a misinformation "infodemic" to proliferate. Specifically, she raises practical considerations on how social media can be leveraged during a pandemic. Complementing the previous chapter, Ken Chen in his chapter "Managing the Spread of Misinformation During COVID-19" (Chapter 10) stresses the importance of understanding the "fear" surrounding the virus, and how, if misunderstood, would drive the spread of misinformation. He also emphasised the need to develop evidence-based strategies to manage the spread of fear and misinformation. On a related note, Jessie Janny Thenarianto in her chapter "Maintaining Cyber Well-Being During a Pandemic" (Chapter 11) explores the challenges that come with cyberspace and technology use during COVID-19, and conceives five strategies that practitioners, policymakers, as well as members of the public can adopt to maintain their cyber well-being. Finally, Damien Cheong and Stephanie Neubronner in their chapter "Crisis Management and Communication During a Pandemic: Some Thoughts" (Chapter 12) opine the need to treat pandemics as a national security challenge so that multi-faceted crises, such as those presented by COVID-19, can then be handled in a manner that ensures a states' civil, economic, social, and psychological defence.

## *Organisational Related Issues*

Section four of the book contains four chapters on issues and strategies that concern organisations. Paul Englert, in his chapter "How to Enhance

Organisation Functioning in a Pandemic: COVID-19 Lessons in Leadership" (Chapter 13), explores the challenges and opportunities for leaders to stress-test their capability to operate in a crisis such as COVID-19. Specifically, he highlights five leadership skills that are necessary for leaders to cultivate and master as they prepare for what will be the inevitable next upheaval. In the chapter "Sustaining Team Morale Amidst a Pandemic: Lessons from COVID-19" (Chapter 14), Minzheng Hou leverages on various psychological theories to identify recommendations on what leaders can do to sustain high team morale during operations, such as those seen in the COVID-19 pandemic. Vivian Seah, John Yu, and Whistine Chai, in their chapter "Telecommuting During a Pandemic: Tips for Parents and Caregivers of the Elderly" (Chapter 15), consolidate the best practices proposed by worldwide experts on how individuals who are working from home can cope with family commitments while doing so. They share five psychological tips that would serve as a meaningful guide for employees to be equally successful at home and in the workforce. The last chapter in this section is dedicated to an often-overlooked issue of ensuring compliance to safe distancing measures from members of the public. Ken Chen, Nur Aisyah, and Shannon Ng, in their chapter "Non-compliance with COVID-19 Safe Distancing Measures: Tips from Crisis Negotiators to De-escalate Situations" (Chapter 16), explain why some people would not comply to safe distancing measures, and identify three strategies that could be used to persuade people to comply peacefully to such measures.

### *Future Directions*

The last chapter "Surviving the Next Pandemic: Lessons for Humanity" (Chapter 17) by Majeed Khader brings the discourse on preparing for the next pandemic, and the relevance of adopting a multidisciplinary approach to mitigate and respond to COVID-19 to a close, by summarising the key lessons from the preceding chapters, as well as highlighting future research directions.

## Conclusion

Amidst the uncertainty engendered by the COVID-19 pandemic, the real danger lies in the way we respond rather than the actual coronavirus itself.

Negative behaviours that were highlighted in the chapters, such as flouting safe distancing measures, spreading fake news, may impact us in ways we may not even be aware of. Hence, there is an urgent need to identify scientifically defensible interventions and approaches to mitigate these issues and enhance our understanding and response to COVID-19 and future pandemics. Hopefully, this book may serve as a starting point for greater discussions and study of this topic, as well as a useful resource guide that readers can use to protect themselves and their loved ones.

In closing, the editors cite Singapore Prime Minister Lee Hsien Loong, who said:

> COVID-19 will remain a problem for a long time yet. It will take at least a year, probably longer, before vaccines become widely available. We will have to learn to live with COVID-19 for the long term, as we have done in the past with other dangerous infectious diseases, like tuberculosis. We also have to get used to new arrangements in our daily lives. We must all adjust the way we live, work and play, so that we can reduce the spread of the virus, and keep ourselves safe. ("In Full: PM Lee's Address," 2020, para. 3).

These comments greatly echo the sentiments of the editors of this book. To safeguard our livelihood and overcome the adversities brought upon by COVID-19, we have to work together for the betterment of the society and to adopt a resilient mindset in order to adapt and thrive in the new unknown.

# References

Bais, A. M. S. (2020). *How psychology can help or hinder the fight against COVID-19*. World Economic Forum. https://www.weforum.org/agenda/2020/05/understanding-emotional-epidemiology-is-key-to-halting-the-spread-of-covid-19/

Balkhi, F., Nasir, A., Zehra, A., Riaz, R., F, B., A, N., A, Z., & R, R. (2020). Psychological and Behavioral Response to the Coronavirus (COVID-19) Pandemic. *Cureus Journal of Medical Science, 12*(5). https://doi.org/10.7759/cureus.7923

Bavel, J. J. V., Baicker, K., Boggio, P. S., Capraro, V., Cichocka, A., Cikara, M., Crockett, M. J., Crum, A. J., Douglas, K. M., Druckman, J. N., Drury, J., Dube, O., Ellemers, N., Finkel, E. J., Fowler, J. H., Gelfand, M., Han, S.,

Haslam, S. A., Jetten, J., ... Willer, R. (2020). Using social and behavioural science to support COVID-19 pandemic response. *Nature Human Behaviour*, *4*(5), 460–471. https://doi.org/10.1038/s41562-020-0884-z

Ghosh, N., & Tan D. W. (2020, April 16). Record race to find Covid-19 vaccine cause for optimism. *The Straits Times*. https://www.straitstimes.com/world/united-states/record-race-to-find-covid-19-vaccine-cause-for-optimism

Goh, Y. H. (2020, June 22). S'poreans donated $90m in first five months of 2020, equal to whole of last year's donations. *The Straits Times*. https://www.straitstimes.com/singapore/singaporeans-donate-90million-in-first-five-months-of-2020-equal-to-whole-of-last-years

Hoof, E. V. (2020). *Lockdown is the world's biggest psychological experiment—And we will pay the price*. https://www.weforum.org/agenda/2020/04/this-is-the-psychological-side-of-the-covid-19-pandemic-that-were-ignoring/

Iacurci, G. (2020, May 19). Unemployment is nearing Great Depression levels. Here's how the eras are similar—and different. *CNBC*. https://www.cnbc.com/2020/05/19/unemployment-today-vs-the-great-depression-how-do-the-eras-compare.html

In full: PM Lee's address on Singapore's post-COVID-19 future, the first in a series of ministerial broadcasts. (2020, June 7). *CNA*. https://www.channelnewsasia.com/news/singapore/covid-19-pm-lee-full-speech-ministrial-broadcasts-12813376

Lai, L. (2020, April 28). Singapore has been ramping up testing for coronavirus to help curb spread. *The Straits Times*. https://www.straitstimes.com/singapore/spore-has-been-ramping-up-testing-for-virus-to-help-curb-spread

Lee, Y. N. (2020, May 26). Singapore plans $23.2 billion fourth stimulus package to support coronavirus-hit economy. *CNBC*. https://www.cnbc.com/2020/05/26/singapore-plans-fourth-stimulus-package-for-coronavirus-hit-economy.html

Rittel, H. W., & Webber, M. M. (1973). Dilemmas in a general theory of planning. *Policy Sciences*, *4*(2), 155–169.

Sing along to Home on April 25 to express thanks to frontline and migrant workers. (2020, April 24). *Today*. https://www.todayonline.com/singapore/sing-along-home-april-25-express-thanks-frontline-and-migrant-workers-0

# Section 1

# Societal Resilience Related Issues

# Chapter 1

# A Journal of the COVID Year: What Can We Learn from Previous Pandemics?

Denise Dillon and Ghee Kian Koh

## Introduction

Many of the behaviours reported since the onset of COVID-19 have been repeated across countries and continents: panic buying, stigmatisation and avoidance, suspicion, and irrationality. For example, who will not recall with some sense of wonder the widespread, COVID-related toilet-paper hoarding phenomenon (e.g., Borbon, 2020; Van Dyke *et al.*, 2020)? It may either perplex or reassure people to know that such behaviours are not as uncommon as we might expect and that similar behaviours have been reported for centuries.

Written in the form of a journal of memoirs, Daniel Defoe's fictional work, *A Journal of the Plague Year*, was published in 1722. Defoe depicts events of the 1664–1665 bubonic plague (also known as the Black Death) as experienced by a merchant in London, known only as H.F. (Defoe, 1722/1986). Worldwide fatalities from the bubonic plague are reported to have been approximately 50 million in the 14th century (Benedictow, 2015); in the 1665–1666 London epidemic alone, almost 15% of the population at that time died from the bubonic plague, with 68,596 deaths recorded in the city over the 18 months (The National Archives UK, n.d.). Healey (2003) describes the Journal as "dynamic history" in that Defoe himself drew on the past "in order to confront the anxieties and mediate and shape the debates of the author's own time" (p. 26). In current times during the COVID-19 pandemic, countries have engaged in debates over ship movement and disembarkation, with reports of up to 100,000 seafarers effectively shipbound due to concerns of potential community transfer of the virus from those onboard (Charles & Okadia, 2020). In Defoe's time, the debate included that of ship quarantine policies and trade embargos on countries in which the plague was also rife. As such, Healey surmises that Defoe may have aligned his fictional account with his government's efforts to sway people's opinions in their favour, and this "journalistic sensationalism" was intended "to convey 'horror' sufficient to 'impress' and 'surprise' people's minds" (p. 26). Of course, our focus is on more recent times, and we have more traditionally objective accounts in the form of peer-reviewed, scholarly literature from which to draw insights and potential guidance, but we also have a plethora of media reports that can so readily influence behaviour just as Defoe's journalistic account did. Some of the more contemporary pandemics experienced in the past decades involved novel infectious diseases such as the SARS coronavirus and the H1N1 virus.

Originating in Guangdong, China, in 2002, SARS was "the first novel infectious disease to emerge in the 21st century" (Sim & Chua, 2004, p. 811). There were 908 fatalities and more than 8,000 people infected in 29 countries as a result of the SARS virus (Teo *et al.*, 2005). Researchers who studied the psychosocial effects of that outbreak focused on feelings such as fear (of contagion), stigmatisation, loneliness, boredom, anger, anxiety, and sense of uncertainty, as well as health-seeking behaviours (e.g., Chua *et al.*, 2004; Grace *et al.*, 2005). Other teams similarly reported fear, worry, and social discrimination (e.g., Zheng *et al.*, 2005). A psychiatric team from Hong Kong reported longer-term effects among recovered SARS patients, including anxiety, insomnia, and depression, as well as recurring memories that disrupted daily functioning (Tsang *et al.*, 2004). A team in Singapore also reported high levels of post-traumatic symptoms in a community healthcare setting (Sim *et al.*, 2010) four months after the first outbreak of SARS in Singapore. In an early response to the COVID-19 pandemic and based on reported findings from previous infectious disease outbreaks, Xiang *et al.* (2020) recommended regular clinical screening for depression, anxiety, and suicidality for healthcare workers in hospitals among several other preventive measures.

Similarly, researchers studying the psychosocial effects of the H1N1 virus, which originated in Mexico in 2009, reported fear of the pandemic, risk avoidance, and health-protective behaviours (e.g., Goodwin *et al.*,

2009). The H1N1 virus is a genetically novel subtype (Centers for Disease Control and Prevention [CDC], 2019b) of the influenza A virus. It was responsible for the 1918 flu pandemic which infected around 500 million people worldwide (about one-third of the world's population at that time), and resulted in an estimated 50 million fatalities (CDC, 2019a).

The recurring focus on fear responses is largely due to the novel nature of these infections from which stems from uncertainty that transcends societal and cultural boundaries, thereby increasing "the level of psychosocial morbidity" (Sim & Chua, 2004, p. 811). However, novelty is not the sole instigator of negative psychosocial responses. Ebola is another serious disease that was first reported in 1976 in Zaire (now the Democratic Republic of the Congo [DRC]), with 46 subsequent outbreaks occurring in various countries from 1976 to 2018 (CDC, 2019c). The CDC reports that "there is currently no antiviral drug licensed by the U.S. Food and Drug Administration (FDA) to treat EVD in people", and the 2018 outbreak in the eastern DRC is ongoing. Despite decades of experience in managing Ebola outbreaks, health anxiety referrals to clinicians reportedly increased during times when Ebola outbreaks featured in mass media coverage (Blakey *et al.*, 2015), even in the absence of an actual outbreak.

With respect to the novel coronavirus, known as COVID-19, which originated in Wuhan, China, in December 2019, it appears that the same psychosocial effects are experienced as for other novel infectious disease outbreaks. As of 30 April 2020, the WHO reported 3,060,443 confirmed cases and 211,025 (6.9%) deaths worldwide, with daily counts adding to the numbers of infected and deaths. In the Western Pacific Region (WPR), which encompasses 27 countries including China and Singapore, the WHO reported 200,586 cases and 7,239 deaths (3.6%) as of 17 June, while in Singapore, there were 40,969 cases and 26 deaths (0.06%) (WHO Regional Office for the Western Pacific [WPRO], 2020c). Singapore's number of infected cases was second highest only to China among the WPR countries, which may lead to an expectation of heightened psychosocial problems (e.g., fear, anxiety, stigmatisation) among Singapore's population.

In his precursory exposition to these 21st century outbreaks, Strong (1990) categorised three types of psychosocial reactions to an epidemic: (1) fear, (2) explanation and moralisation, and (3) action or proposed action (see Figure 1.1). These early reactions to major, fatal epidemics constitute a distinctive psychosocial form of response that Strong named

| FEAR | EXPLANATION & MORALISATION | ACTION or PROPOSED ACTION |
|---|---|---|
| • Waves of individual & collective panic<br>  • Suspicion<br>  • Irrationality<br>  • Stigmatisation (avoidance, segregation, persecution) | • Outburst of interpretation<br>  • as to why the disease has occurred<br>• Rashes of moral controversy<br>  • What could have allowed it? (God? Government?)<br>  • Who is to blame? | • Plagues of competing control strategies<br>  • Aimed at controlling disease itself or controlling further epidemics of fear & social dissolution<br>  • Trade & travel disruptions<br>  • Personal privacy & liberty invaded<br>  • Health education enforced |

Figure 1.1. Strong's (1990) typology of psychosocial epidemic in three forms.

"epidemic psychology", which run in parallel with and can be independent from the reality of the viral epidemic.

Strong (1990) argued that epidemic psychology is not activated by disease outbreaks alone, but rather originates in "some fundamental properties of human society and social action" (p. 250) as an ever-present human characteristic. Social structures such as family and social relationships are vulnerable to sudden changes arising from crises that make additional demands of relatively routinised emotions, attitudes and behaviours through disruption and disorientation.

## Five Key Points Concerning Psychosocial Epidemic

Of course, we must consider that these major fatal epidemics and pandemics have the potential for large-scale fatality over a relatively short term—by definition an "apocalypse". Through major literary critic Laurence Buell, we can better understand how pervasive the rhetoric of apocalypticism is. Apocalyptic rhetoric, says Buell, serves to alert people to global environmental threats by arousing their imagination to a "sense of crisis", through this "master metaphor" (Buell, 1995, p. 285). The idea here is that once people's perceptions become aroused to such threats through evocative works, they may be spurred to action and thereby avoid an actual apocalypse. While Buell focuses on the environmental imagination (the ways that people think about nature and our global environment) and its role in how people can adapt to environmental changes, this idea can be applied to the workings of disease pandemics to improve our understanding of the ways that humans react and behave under these circumstances. Unfortunately, much of what people read concerning viral outbreaks come through the mass media rather than high-level literary works, so that the evocative nature of the content drives less-than-desirable behaviours and can indeed proliferate waves of negative responses such as panic buying (Sim *et al.*, 2020).

Another perspective comes from the tendency to consider ourselves and others as collectives, such as groups, organisations, or even collectives of countries (Wagner-Egger *et al.*, 2011). Collectives serve to reduce uncertainty among laypeople by helping to polarise understanding of various actions through dramatised roles. These often feature in prototypical forms described by Russian folklorist Propp, and Wagner-Egger *et al.*, focused on three of these social representations or media dramatisations: (1) heroes (trustworthy, protective agents or leaders), (2) villains (untrustworthy, with malevolent intent), and (3) victims (to be pitied but also potentially dangerous through lack of personal agency). The following sections draw on Strong's (1990) typology as well as these dramatised roles to consider some of the insights we receive through reports about preparedness, management, and surveillance during some of the past outbreaks as well as during the current COVID-19 pandemic in Singapore.

### *Fear: Waves of Individual and Collective Panic*

> However, I cannot say but it had some effect upon the people, and particularly that, as I said before, they grew more cautious whom they took into their houses, and whom they trusted their lives with. (Defoe, 1722/1986, p. 102).

Early success with detection notwithstanding, Singapore's risk status was elevated as the number of infected cases continued to rise rapidly from May through to June (WHO WPRO, 2020a, 2020b, 2020c). The situation was exacerbated in part due to restrictions on some healthcare services being labelled as non-essential, and therefore not as readily accessible to those in need. Given the alarming rise of reported cases, waves of fear would have been understandable. The initiation of online counselling services (e.g., Goh, 2020; Lim, 2020; Tan, 2020) speaks to the understanding of how necessary such services are in times of crisis. The establishment of a COVID-related helpline to offer support for those experiencing stress or anxiety was a government initiative during challenging times, which reflected the government's understanding of the importance to consider both psychological and physiological well-being of citizens.

Fear certainly stood out as a key factor—indeed, as "a sea of emotions"—in a report by the Registered Nurses Association of Ontario (RNAO), on behalf of healthcare workers who nursed patients with SARS during the 2003 outbreak (RNAO, 2003). Nurses voiced expressions of anxiety and stigma as well as frustration and anger, but they also articulated their commitment and pride in their work. Isolation measures, which included nurses being prevented from leaving their respective SARS units, led to a feeling of being in jail (RNAO, 2003). A lack of suitable and systemic preparedness, and the perceived lack of care for their own well-being led to nurses effectively becoming a disempowered and segregated group—excluded from the "process that creates their social worlds" (Ding *et al.*, 2016)—despite their continued professionalism and commitment.

In their paper on SARS-related social justice issues in Canada and Singapore, Ding *et al.* (2016) noted that "the history of epidemics is one of discrimination, stigmatisation, and political and economic oppression..." (p. 22). In their comparative study of SARS situations in Canada and Singapore, Ding and colleagues revealed that Singapore's efforts to generate widespread public support for medical care workers (MCWs) was markedly positive, whereas MCWs in Canada were subjected to discrimination and avoidance. Singapore's efforts beyond top-down intervention at the governing level were generated through professional associations. Once initiated by the professional associations, grassroots-level support followed. The language at the time was of "war", with references to "battles", being "on the frontline", and to the MCWs having to rely on "defence"—e.g., by wearing masks and other defensive covering—through having "no means to attack" (Ding *et al.*, 2016). In their case study on surveillance strategies in Singapore and with specific reference to public discourse during the 2003 SARS outbreak, Teo *et al.* (2005) indicate that it was perhaps such rhetoric that unified Singaporeans by capturing the public attention and fostering cooperation. On the social justice front, it appears that Singapore performed better than Canada during the SARS outbreak.

However, the segmenting in news reports of daily counts of those affected by COVID-19 in Singapore into Singaporean citizens and Permanent Residents (PR) as opposed to foreign workers ("1,426 new COVID-19", 2020) can unwittingly become an explicit message that foreign workers are "other", which might be interpreted as a national prejudice (e.g., Han, 2020). This divide is further emphasised in regular reports referring to "community cases" (e.g., Lin, 2020) involving citizens and PRs to clearly differentiate those counts from those of affected foreign workers (the "dormitory clusters"). This may unintentionally result in stigmatisation and perceiving the foreign worker "outgroup" as infectious.

### *Explanation and Moralisation: Outburst of Interpretation*

> Next to these public things were the dreams of old women, or, I should say, the interpretation of old women upon other people's dreams; and these put abundance of people even out of their wits. (Defoe, 1722/1986, p. 42).

Western media propagated various allegations of a virology lab accident "cover-up" in Wuhan and highlighted the Asian consumption and trade of wild animals, as possible sources for the origin of COVID-19 (Ghosh, 2020). These allegations were escalated when videos of Asians consuming wild bats was falsely described to have been filmed in China (Palmer, 2020). Privately-circulated stories about the source of both SARS and COVID-19 (both novel types of the coronavirus) continue to propagate as myth, but there have been strong science-based suggestions that the coronavirus originated from bats (Chen *et al.*, 2013). As a result, information that COVID-19 human infection began in China only served to reinforce the biased perception of the seemingly less-hygienic and less-civil practices of the Chinese and other Asians.

Such an interpretation not only distracts from the necessary attention that should be directed towards coping with the pandemic, but also misdirects understanding about the increasing threats from human encroachment of natural habitats and exploitation of wild animals (UNEP, 2016). Here, media dramatisation could villainise the source country of the pandemic. This perspective may also be spread among Singaporeans and may then reinforce any prejudice and blaming of non-Singaporeans living in or frequently visiting Singapore for causing local infections, potentially drawing unnecessary divides among locals and foreigners, instead of forming a united front against the pandemic.

## *Explanation and Moralisation: Rashes of Moral Controversy*

> But when I am speaking of the plague as a distemper arising from natural causes, we must consider it as it was really propagated by natural means; nor is it at all the less a judgement for its being under the conduct of human causes and effects... (Defoe, 1722/1986, p. 204).
>
> ...the sick could infect none but those that came within reach of the sick person; but that one man who may have really received the infection and knows it not, but goes abroad about as a sound person, may give the plague to a thousand people... (Defoe, 1722/1986, p. 206).

Defoe placed the cause of the great plague in the hands of human nature as well as in divine judgment. He also identified those infected but without symptoms as being dangerous infectious agents, just as socialising is cautioned against in current times. In their study on lay perceptions of collectives during the 2009 H1N1 outbreak in Europe, Wagner-Egger *et al.* (2011) argued that the dramatised representations symbolically featuring social collectives as heroes, villains, and victims, helped laypeople comprehend the threats associated with the disease outbreak. According to Strong's epidemic psychology (explanation and moralisation), people have the desire to know who is to blame (the villain) and who is responsible for resolving the matter (the hero). Wagner-Egger *et al.* (2011) noted some ambivalence in the notion of the victim because collectives can, at times, be deemed at least partly responsible for their own predicament.

During the COVID-19 outbreak, health workers around the world have been commonly lauded as heroes, while there have been some attempts to sway lay perceptions of some other collectives from that of either villain or victim to hero. For example, in Singapore, once the numbers of affected foreign workers were seen to rise, the public were encouraged to avoid a perception of the foreign or migrant workers as villains (potential spreaders of disease) or victims (helpless targets of disease) (James, 2020). Some of the media reports of foreign workers as victims veered towards demoting the nation of Singapore from hero (for initial success in detecting and containing the virus spread) to villain (e.g., James, 2020; Mahtani, 2020; Mokhtar, 2020). Conversely, media reports began to promote migrant workers to the group of "unsung heroes" who continued to perform maintenance work and other tasks that so often go unnoticed (Khoury, 2020).

The categorisation of occupations serving essential services to the community during the COVID-19 pandemic has led to a clear perception of heroes in the crisis. More attention has been paid to their sacrifices to maintain a functioning society and face the infectious disease on proverbial frontlines (Tai, 2020). This growing appreciation came as a change from the initial fear and irrational reactions towards the healthcare workers, which had also occurred during the SARS outbreak (Teo *et al.*, 2005). Media coverage of their tireless efforts over several months contributed to the hero status of healthcare and other essential workers, as well as those of various volunteer groups.

While largely in control of the COVID-19 situation, the government's apparent lapse in preparedness for screening in the congested foreign worker dormitories (FWDs) had led to record spikes in infected cases ("1,426 new COVID-19", 2020; "No Singaporeans or permanent residents", 2020). The rhetoric of hero or villain becomes ambiguous as issues regarding persistent systemic marginalisation of migrant workers have been brought into focus again, despite the "gold-class" control of the situation experienced by the local community. Such perceptions can also affect social trust in a crisis, as described by Chong (2006).

The viewing of Singapore itself as potentially untrustworthy has implications for public behaviour, particularly so given the notion of the Singapore government as the caretaker of its populace (Teo *et al.*, 2005). However, if public perception were to shift towards a view of their "caretaker" as villainous, it could lead to increasing acts of defiance. Several reports of people flouting social distancing rules implemented during Singapore's circuit breaker period may be indicative of mistrust or an unwillingness to conform among at least some of the populace, with the specially appointed safe distancing enforcement officers being grouped in the category of villains accused of practising double standards in policing rules for local citizens and expatriate communities (Stolarchuk, 2020).

Taking a lesson from the examination of the MERS outbreak in South Korea in 2015, Ha (2016, p. 234) recommended having all stakeholders—including "business establishments, mass media, schools, and the military"—as co-respondents from the outset, rather than having each entity act "as outsiders in a national crisis". Teo *et al.* (2005) also emphasised the importance of gaining public buy-in, even if exercised as compliance, as they concluded was the case in Singapore during the 2003 SARS outbreak. The RNAO report (2003) and Ding *et al.* (2016) reiterate the necessity of a unified response to effect adequate preparedness for responses to future epidemics. Going a step further, and based on their study of psychosocial factors predicting preventive behaviours in SARS-affected regions, Cheng and Ng (2006) recommended addressing future outbreaks at a global level, using a multinational approach involving governments and healthcare professionals from different countries.

### Action: Plagues of Competing Control Strategies

> In a word, they could consider of separating the people into smaller bodies, and removing them in time farther from one another—and not let such a contagion as this, which is indeed chiefly dangerous to collected bodies of people, find a million of people in a body together, as was very near the case before, and would certainly be the case if it should ever happen again. (Defoe, 1722/1986, p. 209).

While so many of us queried one or more of the preventative control measures enacted to reduce the spread of COVID-19, our concerns again are a mirror of people who experienced the great plague. Defoe described a number of measures and roles that, in their familiarity, are surprisingly current, with the "shutting up of houses" as one of the first methods taken, followed by the appointment of examiners, watchmen, and searchers whose roles were to keep people apart from each other, loosely akin to the appointments of safe distancing officers during COVID-19.

Owing to lessons learned from the 2003 SARS experience, protocols, and infrastructures were developed to meet the challenge of future epidemics, but the escalating threat of COVID-19 has already exceeded that of SARS. A limited lockdown, termed the "circuit breaker", was singularly imposed nationwide by the Singapore government for eight weeks, where businesses deemed "non-essential" were asked to cease face-to-face operations and to conduct regular activities remotely if possible (Ministry of Health Singapore, 2020a). This preventive strategy was implemented following an increase in the community spread of infections and growing clusters of infected cases among FWDs (Griffiths, 2020). The non-negotiable policies implemented are reminiscent of the stringent policies enforced to limit the spread of SARS (Teo *et al.*, 2005), which quelled fears of an uncontrollable outbreak and helped cement public trust in the government to lead Singapore through and out of COVID-19. Some ways that the preventive measures have affected the public were identified by Strong (1990) as plagues of competing control strategies: trade and travel disruptions, personal privacy and liberty invaded, and health education enforced.

Compared to SARS, the travel ban in light of COVID-19 was not just informal or limited to certain foreign visitors; instead, complete border closures were ordered in Singapore and most other countries around the world (Ramchandani, 2020). Commercial flights were halted indefinitely, and the causeway crossings between Singapore and Malaysia were also closed. There were no notions of exceptionalism in terms of quarantine periods this time; all who returned to Singapore before border closure were expected to serve a 14-day "stay-home notice" (SHN), with non-compliance by anyone being a legally punishable offence (Ministry of Health Singapore, 2020b). It seems that the gravity of COVID-19 was well-understood to be unprecedented even among those having experienced SARS, but strong leadership is necessary to help individuals understand the sacrifices that needed to be made, and to prevent the society from spiralling into an epidemic of fear and social dissolution simultaneously.

Invasions of personal privacy and liberty took similar forms in Singapore as for Defoe's plague-infested London, with bans on gatherings of people beyond their households as well as restrictions on access to public eating places and the closure of entertainment establishments. During the COVID-19 outbreak, Singapore's residents were expected to comply with SHN and quarantine orders as deemed necessary, with less-intrusive means of ensuring compliance as technology advanced in the years since SARS. The use of video-calling functions on smartphones has negated the need for installing cameras in private lodgings that might have felt more intrusive during the SARS period (Teo *et al.*, 2005). Contact tracing technology has also been refined with the utilisation of Bluetooth-based personal smartphone applications (Aravindan & Phartiyal, 2020), although the uptake of such tracing apps among the public was lower than desired, which may indicate public resistance to intrusion on personal privacy, although other explanations are possible. According to Teo *et al.* (2005, p. 290), "The SARS episode revealed that compliance is effective and necessary for the containment of infectious diseases". Circuit breaker measures compromised liberty for all people but were accepted with reasonable compliance as was the case during the SARS outbreak. This may very well be due to a continuing "crisis mentality" among the Singapore population as argued by Teo *et al.* (2005); however, we must consider that perceived compliance may also be in part due to the presently ill-defined construct of risk perception (Leppin & Aro, 2009). For example, what some might consider to be health-protective behaviours based on risk perceptions might instead be founded on cognitively driven outcome expectancies (cost-benefit considerations). For example, people may be motivated more by concerns about what they stand to lose in terms of economic or national stability than by perceptions of any threat posed by a disease. Further, motivation to engage in protective behaviours may depend on whether the focus is on the expectancy component (the likelihood of contracting a disease) or on the value component (how severely might the disease affect me) (Leppin & Aro, 2009).

The enforcement of health education in Singapore during the SARS outbreak was predominantly managed through authoritative sources. As with international acclamation for efforts in the early stages of COVID-19, during the SARS outbreak, Singapore was lauded for its "open and responsive risk communication" (Dr. Peter Sandman, as cited in Chong, 2006). In particular, Tan Tock Seng Hospital won the International Public Relations Society's Gold Award in acknowledgement of their engagement in communication to promote public awareness and encourage public surveillance (Chong, 2006). In the current COVID-19 outbreak, a government-based messaging service was initiated for constant communication, demonstrating recognition of the importance of open communication that had been elaborated by Chong (2006).

Such success notwithstanding, the conceptual understanding of risk perception itself has come under scrutiny in terms of what risk is and what determines risk perception (Leppin & Aro, 2009). In his paper recommending some lessons to be learned from the SARS epidemic, Chong (2006) noted that "social and psychological impacts are disproportionate to the relatively low global mortality rates associated with the disease" (p. 6). If risk communication is to be truly effective, stakeholders should be clear about the nature of risk and how components of risk are perceived (e.g., cognitively, emotionally, or both cognitive and emotional). In addition, such clear communication is especially vital when facing a novel pandemic such as COVID-19, where our understanding of the virus develops and changes over time. The formation of risk perceptions is another issue that Leppin and Aro (2009) underscored for further clarification, and particularly so with respect to infectious diseases due to the social basis of transmission, which thereby extends risk perception beyond the self but also to close and more distant others.

## *Proposed Action: Aimed at Controlling Further Epidemics of Fear and Social Dissolution*

Taken together, it becomes evident that a number of lessons were learned through experiences of managing the SARS epidemic in Singapore, although it is also evident that Singapore was ahead of many other countries even at that time in terms of effective management strategies.

1.  *Waves of fear and seas of emotion*: Managing the rhetoric; positive messages encompassing groups at all levels of society; avoiding easy categorisation of outgroups—"all in it together".
2.  *Outbursts of interpretation*: Early and clear messages about the origin and nature of the disease.
3.  *Rashes of moral controversy*: Combined efforts across borders: combat marginalisation and adopt social justice perspective for all, plus the importance of being prepared—the hero factor.
4.  *Plagues of competing control strategies*: Consider the nature of risk perception and compliance, as well as other drivers of human behaviour in times of crisis when circumstances can change rapidly.

# Conclusion

Strong (1990) proposed that the characteristics of his epidemic psychology model are "a permanent part of the human condition" (p. 249). Whatever his motivation, Defoe (1722/1986) managed to capture each of the elements of psychosocial epidemic (fear, explanation and moralisation, action or proposed action) centuries prior to Strong (1990) having the opportunity to develop his typology, which at least speaks to the enduring nature of epidemic psychology. Just as Defoe (1722/1986) constructed accounts of individual and collective panic among London city dwellers at the onset and throughout the duration of the great plague, current reports narrate incidents of fear-driven behaviours, outbursts of interpretation, and rashes of moral controversy, as well as plagues of competing control strategies. While some of the more prominent occurrences were in other countries, the Singaporean population was nonetheless influenced to some extent in the reporting and interpretation of such events through local and personal channels of communication. Given the carefully curated series of strategic preventative measures implemented by the Singaporean government, it becomes evident that responses were aligned not only with what has occurred in the past, but also with an eye to the future.

Fortunately, the worst of such apocalyptic events have still been kept at bay, due to the preparedness derived from the SARS experience. The decisive leadership of the Singapore government and community support from the people are other factors underlying successful crisis management. However, the need to prevent a further psychosocial epidemic continues as the economy reopens following the circuit breaker. Support for the unemployed and marginalised, improved wages for underpaid essential workers, and the improvement of living conditions for migrant workers will be closely observed, which can determine if the people's trust in the government and its leadership will remain.

# References

1,426 new COVID-19 cases in Singapore, mostly foreign workers in dormitories. (2020, April 21). *Channel News Asia.* https://www.channelnewsasia.com/news/singapore/covid-19-new-cases-1426-foreign-workers-dormitory-citizen-pr-moh-12658250

Aravindan, A., & Phartiyal, S. (2020, April 21). Bluetooth phone apps for tracking COVID-19 show modest early results. *Reuters.* https://www.reuters.com/article/us-health-coronavirus-apps/bluetooth-phone-apps-for-tracking-covid-19-show-modest-early-results-idUSKCN2232A0

Benedictow, O. (2015, March 3). The Black Death: The greatest catastrophe ever. *History Today.* https://www.historytoday.com/archive/black-death-greatest-catastrophe-ever

Blakey, S. M., Reuman, L., Jacoby, R. J., & Abramowitz, J. S. (2015). Tracing "Fearbola": Psychological predictors of anxious responding to the threat of Ebola. *Cognitive Therapy and Research, 39,* 816–825. https://doi.org/10.1007/s10608-015-9701-9

Borbon, C. (2020, March 17). Coronavirus panic buying: The psychology behind toilet paper hoarding. *Gulf News.* https://gulfnews.com/photos/news/coronavirus-panic-buying-the-psychology-behind-toilet-paper-hoarding-1

Buell, L. (1995). *The Environmental Imagination: Thoreau, Nature Writing, and the Formation of American Culture.* Belknap Press of Harvard University Press.

Centers for Disease Control and Prevention. (2019a, March 20). *1918 Pandemic.* https://www.cdc.gov/flu/pandemic-resources/1918-pandemic-h1n1.html

Centers for Disease Control and Prevention. (2019b, June 11). *2009 H1N1 Pandemic (H1N1pdm09 virus).* https://www.cdc.gov/flu/pandemic-resources/2009-h1n1-pandemic.html

Centers for Disease Control and Prevention. (2019c, November 5). *Ebola (Ebola Virus Disease).* https://www.cdc.gov/vhf/ebola/index.html

Charles, C., & Okadia, D. (2020, May 5). Uncharted waters Of COVID-19 quarantine: What is next for seafarers after repatriation? *Marine Insight.* https://www.marineinsight.com/shipping-news/uncharted-waters-of-covid-19-quarantine-what-is-next-for-seafarers-after-repatriation/

Chen, F., Cao, S., Xin, J., & Luo, X. (2013). Ten years after SARS: Where was the virus from? *Journal of Thoracic Disease, 5*(2), 163–167. https://doi.org/10.3978/j.issn.2072-1439.2013.06.09

Cheng, C., & Ng, A. K. (2006). Psychosocial Factors Predicting SARS-Preventive Behaviors in Four Major SARS-Affected Regions. *Journal of Applied Social Psychology, 36*(1), 222–247. https://doi.org/10.1111/j.0021-9029.2006.00059.x

Chong, M. (2006). A crisis of epidemic proportions: What communication lessons can practitioners learn from the Singapore SARS crisis? *Public Relations Quarterly, 51*(1), 6–11. https://ink.library.smu.edu.sg/lkcsb_research/2480/

Chua, S. E., Cheung, V., McAlonan, G. M., Cheung, C., Wong, J. W. S., Cheung, E. P. T., Chan, M. T., Wong, T. K., Choy, K. M., Chu, C. M., Lee, P. W., & Tsang, K. W. T. (2004). Stress and psychological impact on SARS patients during the outbreak. *Canadian Journal of Psychiatry, 49*(6), 385–390. https://doi.org/10.1177/070674370404900607

Defoe, D. (1722/1986). *A journal of the plague year: Being observations or memorials of the most remarkable occurrences, as well public as private, which happened in London during the last great visitation in 1665. Written by a citizen who continued all the while in London. Never made public before.* (A. Burgess & C. Bristow, Eds.). Penguin Books.

Ding, H., Li, X., & Haigler, A. C. (2016). Access, oppression, and social (in)justice in epidemic control: Race, profession, and communication in SARS outbreak in Canada and Singapore. *English Faculty Publications, 111.* https://doi.org/10.21310/cnx.4.1.16dinetal

Ghosh, N. (2020, May 7). China, US stand-off over origin of COVID-19 deepens. *The Straits Times.* https://www.straitstimes.com/world/united-states/china-us-standoff-over-origin-of-covid-19-deepens

Goh, T. (2020, April 11). Coronavirus: Free teleconsultations for those in need of mental health support. *The Straits Times*. https://www.straitstimes.com/singapore/health/free-teleconsultations-for-those-in-need-of-mental-health-support

Goodwin, R., Haque, S., Neto, F., & Myers, L. B. (2009). Initial psychological responses to Influenza A, H1N1 ("Swine flu"). *BMC Infectious Diseases, 9*, 166. https://doi.org/10.1186/1471-2334-9-166

Grace, S. L., Hershenfield, K., Robertson, E., & Stewart, D. E. (2005). The occupational and psychosocial impact of SARS on academic physicians in three affected hospitals. *Psychosomatics, 46*(5), 385–391. https://doi.org/10.1176/appi.psy.46.5.385

Griffiths, J. (2020, April 19). Singapore had a model coronavirus response, then cases spiked. *CNN*. https://edition.cnn.com/2020/04/18/asia/singapore-coronavirus-response-intl-hnk/index.html

Ha, K. M. (2016). A lesson learned from the MERS outbreak in South Korea in 2015. *Journal of Hospital Infection, 9*, 232–234. https://dx.doi.org/10.1016%2Fj.jhin.2015.10.004

Han, K. (2020, May 16). Singapore is trying to forget migrant workers are people. The outbreak in crowded dorms has brought out the city-state's prejudices. *FP Insider Access*. https://foreignpolicy.com/2020/05/06/singapore-coronavirus-pandemic-migrant-workers/

Healy, M. (2003). Defoe's Journal and the English plague writing tradition. *Literature and Medicine, 22*(1), 25–44. https://doi.org/10.1353/lm.2003.0006

James, C. (2020, May 8). Singapore must rethink how it treats migrant workers. Coronavirus outbreak highlights poor pay, crowded dormitories and prejudice. *Nikkei Asian Review*. https://asia.nikkei.com/Opinion/Singapore-must-rethink-how-it-treats-migrant-workers

Khoury, N. (2020, April 11). How to help migrant workers affected by COVID-19 in Singapore. *SG Lifestyle*. https://www.buro247.sg/lifestyle/news/how-to-help-migrant-workers-affected-by-covid19-in-singapore.html

Leppin, A., & Aro, A. R. (2009). Risk Perceptions Related to SARS and Avian Influenza: Theoretical Foundations of Current Empirical Research. *International Journal of Behavioral Medicine, 16*(1), 7–29. https://doi.org/10.1007/s12529-008-9002-8

Lim, Y. L. (2020, April 5). Government to set up Covid-19 hotline offering emotional support, CCs and RCs to close from Tuesday. *The Straits Times*. https://www.straitstimes.com/singapore/government-to-set-up-covid-19-hotline-offering-emotional-support

Lin, J. (2020, May 21). Singapore is nearing 30,000 in Covid-19 cases—and the number of Singaporeans/PRs just jumped to 13. *MSN*. https://www.msn.com/en-sg/news/singapore/singapore-is-nearing-30000-in-covid-19-cases-and-the-number-of-singaporeans-prs-just-jumped-to-13/ar-BB14peWt

Mahtani, S. (2020, April 21). Singapore lost control of its coronavirus outbreak, and migrant workers are the victims. *Washington Post.* https://www. washingtonpost.com/world/2020/04/21/singapore-lost-control-its-coronavirus-outbreak-migrant-workers-are-victims/?arc404=true

Ministry of Health Singapore. (2020a, April 14). *Continued stringent implementation & enforcement of circuit breaker measures.* https://www. moh.gov.sg/news-highlights/details/continued-stringent-implementation-enforcement-of-circuit-breaker-measures

Ministry of Health Singapore. (2020b, March 15). *Additional precautionary measures to prevent further importation of COVID-19 cases.* https://www. moh.gov.sg/news-highlights/details/additional-precautionary-measures-to-prevent-further-importation-of-covid-19-cases

Mokhtar, F. (2020, April 21). How Singapore flipped from virus hero to cautionary tale. *Bloomberg News.* https://www.bloomberg.com/news/articles/2020-04-21/how-singapore-flipped-from-virus-hero-to-cautionary-tale

No Singaporeans or permanent residents among the 373 new COVID-19 cases in Singapore. (2020, May 28). *Channel News Asia.* https://www.channelnewsasia. com/news/singapore/covid-19-may-28-no-new-singapore-citizen-pr-cases-373-12778182

Palmer, J. (2020, January 27). Don't blame bat soup for the coronavirus. *Foreign Policy.* https://foreignpolicy.com/2020/01/27/coronavirus-covid19-dont-blame-bat-soup-for-the-virus/

Ramchandani, N. (2020, March 22). Singapore to shut borders to short term visitors from Monday, 11.59pm. *The Business Times.* https://www. businesstimes.com.sg/government-economy/singapore-to-shut-borders-to-short-term-visitors-from-monday-1159pm

RNAO. (2003). SARS Unmasked. *A report on the Nursing Experience with SARS in Ontario Presented to the Commission to Investigate the Introduction and Spread of SARS in Ontario Public Hearing: September 29, 2003.* http://www.archives.gov.on.ca/en/e_records/sars/hearings/01Mon.pdf/Mon_10_45_RNAO.pdf

Sim, K., Chan, Y. H., Chong, P. N., Chua, H. C., & Soon, S. W. (2010). Psychosocial and coping responses within the community health care setting towards a national outbreak of an infectious disease. *Journal of Psychosomatic Research, 68*(2), 195–202. https://doi.org/10.1016/j. jpsychores.2009.04.004

Sim, K., & Chua, H. C. (2004). The psychological impact of SARS: A matter of heart and mind. *Canadian Medical Association Journal, 170*(5), 811–812. https://dx.doi.org/10.1503%2Fcmaj.1032003

Sim, K., Chua, H. C., Vieta, E., & Fernandez, G. (2020). Letter to the Editor: The anatomy of panic buying related to the current COVID-19 pandemic.

*Psychiatry Research, 288,* 113015. https://doi.org/10.1016/j.psychres.2020. 113015

Stolarchuk, J. (2020, May 18). Questions of double standards arise as expat crowds gather freely at Robertson Quay. *The Independent.* http://theindependent.sg/questions-of-double-standards-arise-as-expat-crowds-gather-freely-at-robertson-quay/

Strong, P. (1990). Epidemic psychology: A model. *Sociology of Health & Illness, 12*(3), 249–259. https://doi.org/10.1111/1467-9566.ep11347150

Tai, J. (2020, June 14). 8 in 10 Singaporeans willing to pay more for essential services: Survey. *The Straits Times.* https://www.straitstimes.com/singapore/manpower/8-in-10-singaporeans-willing-to-pay-more-for-essential-services

Tan, T. (2020). All stressed out by Covid-19 outbreak? Keep calm, free online counselling is at hand. *The Straits Times.* https://www.straitstimes.com/singapore/all-stressed-out-by-covid-19-outbreak-keep-calm-free-online-counselling-is-at-hand

Teo, P., Yeoh, B. S. A., & Ong, S. N. (2005). SARS in Singapore: Surveillance strategies in a globalising city. *Health Policy, 72,* 279–291. https://doi.org/10.1016/j.healthpol.2004.11.004

The National Archives UK. (n.d.). *Great Plague of 1665–1666.* https://www.nationalarchives.gov.uk/education/resources/great-plague/

Tsang, H. W. H., Scudds, R. J., & Chan, E. Y. L. (2004). Psychosocial impact of SARS. *Emerging Infectious Diseases, 10*(7), 1326–1327. https://dx.doi.org/10.3201/eid1007.040090

UNEP. (2016). *UNEP Frontiers 2016 Report: Emerging Issues of Environmental Concern.* https://environmentlive.unep.org/media/docs/assessments/UNEP_Frontiers_2016_report_emerging_issues_of_environmental_concern.pdf

Van Dyke, M., Carusa, S., & Warren, T. (2020). *Understanding Hoarding Responses to Covid-19: Where Did All the Toilet Paper Go?* Anxiety and Depression Association of America. https://adaa.org/learn-from-us/from-the-experts/blog-posts/consumer/understanding-hoarding-responses-covid-19-where

Wagner-Egger, P., Bangerter, A., Gilles, I., Green, E., Rigaud, D., Krings, F., Staerklé, C., & Clémence, A. (2011). Lay perceptions of collectives at the outbreak of the H1N1 epidemic: Heroes, villains and victims. *Public Understanding of Science, 20*(4), 461–476. https://doi.org/10.1177/0963662510393605

WHO Regional Office for the Western Pacific (WPRO). (2020a, May 27). *COVID-19 Situation Report for the Western Pacific Region* (External Situation Report #4). https://www.who.int/westernpacific/internal-publications-detail/covid-19-situation-report-for-the-western-pacific-region-04-20-may-2020---26-may-2020

WHO Regional Office for the Western Pacific (WPRO). (2020b, June 10). *Coronavirus Disease 2019 (COVID-19)* (External Situation Report #6). https://www.who.int/westernpacific/internal-publications-detail/covid-19-situation-report-for-the-western-pacific-region-06-3-june-2020---9-june-2020

WHO Regional Office for the Western Pacific (WPRO). (2020c, June 17). *Coronavirus Disease 2019 (COVID-19)* (External Situation Report #7). https://www.who.int/westernpacific/internal-publications-detail/covid-19-situation-report-for-the-western-pacific-region-07-10-june-2020---16-june-2020

Xiang, Y.-T., Yang, Y., Li, W., Zhang, L., Zhang, Q., Cheung, T., & Ng, C. H. (2020). Timely mental health care for the 2019 novel coronavirus outbreak is urgently needed. *The Lancet Psychiatry, 7*(3), 228–229. https://doi.org/10.1016/s2215-0366(20)30046-8

Zheng, G., Jimba, M., & Wakai, S. (2005). Exploratory study on psychosocial impact of the severe acute respiratory syndrome (SARS) outbreak on Chinese students living in Japan. *Asia Pacific Journal of Public Health, 17*(2), 124–129. https://doi.org/10.1177/101053950501700211

# Chapter 2

# What are the Economic Impacts of a Pandemic?

Jose M. L. Montesclaros

## Introduction: The Pandemic Paradox

A pandemic is defined by the World Health Organisation as a "worldwide spread of a new disease" with evidenced potential to create significant harm to communities (World Health Organisation [WHO], 2010). The declaration of COVID-19 as a pandemic sent strong signals to countries to start taking the disease seriously, and to apply whatever measures that are required, including lockdown policies. The paradox, though, is that any disease is potentially a pandemic, but no matter how infectious or lethal it is, it can only be declared as a pandemic after it has spread through infections to multiple countries globally.

Along the way, the WHO had discouraged countries from shutting down airports to minimise unnecessary economic losses from the disease (Nebehay, 2020), and even said that people who were feeling well did not need to wear masks (Naftulin, 2020). In fact, by mid-February, it was thought that the virus had already started to wind down, with new lab-confirmed cases per day going down from approximately 4,000 on 5 February to 1,000 on 16 February; at this time, there were a total of 51,857 cases and under 2,000 deaths, mostly in China (WHO, 2020a). COVID-19 was eventually declared as a pandemic on 11 March 2020, more than three months since its emergence. By this time, it had already planted its seed in more than 100 countries, infecting 118,000 and killing more than 4,000 people (WHO, 2020b). As countries saw their infection rates rising, governments eventually started to implement quarantine policies to arrest COVID-19's spread.

Fast forward to today, it is easy to see that the policy advice allowed by the evidence at that time had led global society to grossly under-estimate the potential impact that the pandemic could cause, with 4.7 million cases globally, and over 315,000 deaths as of 18 May (Worldometer, 2020). In fact, news reports have shown that the COVID-19 pandemic does not choose its victims according to wealth or status, whether it be the United Kingdom's Prime Minister Boris Johnson, Monaco's Prince Albert II, Russia's Prime Minister Mikhail Mishustin, or the United States Senator Rand Paul ("Coronavirus Pandemic", 2020). Moreover, its potential to develop into an economic crisis led the International Monetary Fund (IMF) to refer to today's situation as "The Great Lockdown", a play of words referencing the Great Depression of the 1930s (IMF, 2020a).

This chapter explains the economic impacts of today's lockdown policies. It first discusses how the pandemic affects some economic sectors, detailing the primary channels of impact. It then describes the dynamics of how such economic disruptions can spiral into economic crises, based on the behaviour of aggregate producers and spenders. It also highlights how poorer individuals carry a larger share of the burden, and how the failure to address their needs could potentially lead to protests/disorder. Next, it explains the logic behind the interventions taken by governments to prevent a downward spiral into a crisis, and the need to help countries who are already in debt distress in order to give them the leeway to enact the needed healthcare spending as well as support to businesses. This chapter ends on a positive note by highlighting how increased government support and international cooperation that is present today, could spell a different outcome and trend of recovery from the previous 2007–2008 Global Financial Crisis.

## How a Pandemic Impacts the Economic Sector

Lockdowns are the key modes of transmission from "pandemic" to "economic crisis". This section explains the relationship by highlighting COVID-19's elusive nature of "asymptomatic transmission" as the rationale for lockdowns, as well as its novelty as the basis for why lockdowns are protracted.

## Risk of Asymptomatic Transmission: Rationale for Lockdowns

An important trait about the COVID-19 virus is that a person can show no symptoms and yet be able to infect others through droplets, or asymptomatic transmission (Gandhi *et al.*, 2020). This makes standard temperature test for fevers an unreliable assessment for the presence of the virus. Due to this elusive nature, anyone who has ever interacted with another person should act as if they had contracted the virus, by wearing masks to prevent them from infecting others. At the same time, they must also act as if they did not have it, by practicing social distancing to avoid contracting it.

The uncertainty brought about by the pandemic's trait of contagiousness even in the absence of symptoms, is at the crux of its economic impact. The only way to definitively contain it is to reduce the probability of physical contact, through the implementation of quarantine measures, also known as "lockdowns", "circuit breakers", or "community quarantines" (WHO, 2020c). Given these traits of the virus, the IMF speculated in April 2020 that the pandemic could cause a 3% reduction in global gross domestic product (GDP), which is significantly worse than the previous 2007–2008 financial crisis (IMF, 2020a).

## Novelty of the Virus

COVID-19's economic impact is aggravated by its novel nature, which extends the amount of time required for finding a vaccine or cure. This, in turn, requires a longer period of lockdown. As of late-May 2020, more than five months since the virus first emerged in December 2019, no vaccine or cure has yet been recommended for general use.

In an updated report in May 2020, the Asian Development Bank (ADB) hinged its estimates of COVID-19's economic impacts on the duration of global lockdowns. If lockdowns lasted three months, then the worst-case scenario was a shrinkage of 6.4%, and if it were to last six months, it would be 9.7% (ADB, 2020a). Based on these scenarios, ADB forecasted that between 158 and 242 million individuals would be laid off, and that total wage income would fall by USD1.2 trillion to USD1.8 trillion (ADB, 2020a).

Some have argued that the duration of quarantines should be weighed against the economic losses they bring to society whenever cities are locked down, to the point of putting dollar values to lives and comparing these to livelihoods lost (Quah & Swee, 2020). However, this can be contested on both ethical and logical grounds. The priority of governments is to protect the lives of their citizens. Moreover, contracting COVID-19 does not necessarily equate to death. Instead, the link between infection and death depends significantly on the availability of hospital capacity to accommodate COVID-19 patients, as well as the availability of vaccines and/or treatments. Therefore, safe distancing measures will need to be put in place until a vaccine is found. Moreover, a key consideration in opening up, is whether there is sufficient hospital capacity to address new cases.

# Primary Channels of Impact

The forecasted contraction of 6% to 9% (ADB, 2020a) can be understood intuitively, if one envisions a "circular economy" wherein companies and consumers interact with one another to determine price levels, and in turn, employment and wages. From this perspective, COVID-19's effects on national GDP can be measured as the sum of its effects on the multiple sectors or industries that make up the economy.

### Sectors Affected by Travel Bans

The first types of economic effects of COVID-19 occurred when countries shut their borders to travel and tourism. Initially, when it was perceived as a "China disease", the estimates by the ADB focused on the effects of reduced demand from the country that was on its way to become the world's largest economy. Even in its worst-case scenario, the impact was only 2% reduction in China's consumption levels, with secondary effects of 50% reduced outbound tourism from China that impacted countries, which have imposed travel bans against China (ADB, 2020b). Today, all countries having imposed mutual travel bans on one another, can be expected to experience the same impacts of COVID-19, with the cancellation of many international events, and in turn, flights, hotel, and restaurant bookings, among others (Elliott, 2020).

### Sectors Affected by Lockdowns

The second types of economic effects of COVID-19 occurred when countries impose domestic lockdowns. These focus mostly on "non-essential" goods and services. The halting of non-essential services should not be underestimated, given that even if they are not considered to be essential, they still contribute significantly to the economy.

At a time when there is significant income inequality and where approximately 10% of the world live below the poverty line, non-essential goods and services are primarily consumed by the majority 90% who are not poor. Therefore, a key driver of GDP contraction will be through the closure of such manufacturing factories. For instance, non-essential goods include manufacturing of industrial equipment, which accounts for 25% of global GDP and 30% of employment (Accenture, 2020). This also impacts other services, such as restaurants, gyms, furniture, cosmetics, travel, tourism, and non-essential medical services.

## International Spill-over Effects from Countries with Deficient Health Systems

The effects of travel bans and lockdowns can have further spill-over effects, given the interlinked nature of supply chains. This may prevent firms providing essential goods and services from operating at their peak levels, given that essential industries rely on non-essential industries for their tools and supplies, without which they cannot operate.

At the international level, the exposure of supply chains to disruption depending on whether they are located in countries who are strongly affected by COVID-19. According to an article in the *Harvard Business Review*, even if production costs may be lower in China, the increased economic risk arising from health sector vulnerabilities, have led to talks of an "Exodus from China" on the part of companies headquartered in major economies, such as the United States, Canada, countries in Europe, and Australia (Govindarajan & Bagla, 2020).

Today, these effects are not exclusive to China, as other countries have been equally affected, and moving forward, many countries are equally vulnerable to the emergence of the same types of health risk. According to the Economist Intelligence Unit's report and webinar released in October 2019, no country today is prepared for a new pandemic, with an average score of less than 50 out of 100 in global health security and preparedness (Economist Intelligence Unit, 2019).

## Spill-over Effects from the Transport Sector

A further spill-over effect, whether internationally or domestically, is through the transport sector—i.e., logistics, marketing, and distribution.

This sector can be hindered from operating at normal levels, whether because of illness and death of employees, or because of quarantine policies that prevent employees from going to work.

By limiting the deliveries and transactions that can be made within a country, the impact of transport sector disruptions has affected the supply chains. For instance, if the transport sector is not operating at full capacity (e.g., 90%), this practically reduces the number of transactions or extent of economic activity that can be performed. This is evidenced by supply-chain gluts in the energy sector, such as meeting the full capacity for oil tanks in China's docks (Xu *et al.*, 2020). In the food sector, the inability of farmers to access feeds for growing livestock, is causing a slowdown in the production of pork, which leads to increase in domestic prices (Bermingham, 2020).

## How Economic Impacts Can Spiral Into Economic Crises: Behavioural Risks

Not all economic disruptions lead to economic crises. For instance, production activities in economic sectors have been affected in the past by diseases, such as Avian Influenza or Swine Influenza, when chickens or swine were required to be culled, or by natural disasters that destroy infrastructure. However, these disruptions did not always lead to crises; for the most part, they could be contained within the affected economic sectors.

For a disruption to evolve into a crisis, the economic impact should be both severe and long-lasting. Interestingly, it is not so much the physical or temporal impact of disruptions that cause crises, as it is how disruptions influence the psychology of producers and consumers. Keynesian economics, which guides counter-cyclical government policies today to prevent crises, assumes this. This began with the recognition that the Great Depression of the 1930s was the result of a problem in coordinating the expectations among producers, and between producers and consumers. In today's pandemic, two conditions need to be met for the impacts described above to spiral into a crisis.

### *Step One: Producers Cut Production Targets*

On the producers' side, the economic logic is rather straightforward from a business point of view—they do not wish to produce more than they can sell. They may reduce their production levels over an extended period of time, if they expect that there will be less demand (given job/income disruptions), or that the controls on the movement of people and transport disruptions will prevent them from reaching their markets. If they do not engage in such behaviours, they risk spoilage of unsold goods (with short shelf-lives), or having to pay higher costs for storing them.

### Step Two: Producers Cut Down Workers or Salaries

Next, when companies reduce their production targets, it implies that they cannot hire as many workers as they do during normal operations; otherwise, they would incur greater financial losses from lower levels of productivity. At a time when access to overseas markets is limited because of the lockdowns in their partner countries in trade, the key consumers they will be the very same people who earn salaries from employment.

Thus, if all producers within locked down economies decide to cut back on wages or employment, then the same producers will suffer from further reductions in sales and revenues, beyond the reductions in sales that would have occurred from the lockdowns per se. While it is ideal for firms not to cut employment or reduce wages, it is also important to note that for some firms, this is not a matter of choice. Small- and medium-sized enterprises (SMEs), which make up over 90% of all businesses in the Asia Pacific, are not likely to hold sufficient capital to be able to pay the same amount of wages during the disruption (UNESCAP, 2012).

### Downward Spiral into Recession and Crisis

This sequence of events, therefore, is what can trigger economies to spiral down into recessions, and possibly depressions—which are more severe and protracted. The ADB projected that global trade—including both imports and exports—may shrink by USD1.7 to 2.6 trillion, according to their three- and six-month scenarios (ADB, 2020a). With less/no income, the appetite and capacity of these buyers to purchase products will also be significantly reduced. The ADB has also forecasted a USD1.2 to 1.8 trillion reduction in wages, with over 158 to 242 million individuals losing their jobs (ADB, 2020a). The International Labour Organisation estimated the share of global employment at risk to be 37.5%, and it can be broken down into the following: "food and accommodation (144 million workers), retail and wholesale (482 million), business services and administration (157 million), and manufacturing (463 million)" ("COVID-19: Impact", 2020, para. 5).

## Worse Effects on Vulnerable Groups, and the Potential for Protests/Disorder

Some members of society carry a larger share of the burden of the COVID-19 pandemic. According to the ADB, COVID-19 could potentially lead 200 to 400 million more individuals into poverty—based on the USD3.2 per day poverty line (ADB, 2020a). Further analysis by the International Food Policy Research Institute estimates that a global economic slowdown of 1% translates to a 2% increase in global poverty rates, majority of which—approximately 64%—are in rural areas (Debucquet & Martin, 2018; Vos *et al.*, 2020). Beyond these, this section elaborates on the pandemic's impacts within urban settings.

### *Limited Job Demand During Lockdowns*

The most significant impact for middle-to-upper class individuals may be that they need to work from home and forego their usual consumption habits, such as shopping for consumer goods or services (e.g., haircuts). In the case of the lower-income group, who live from hand-to-mouth and do not have savings to tap onto, the inability to work means that they may not be able to meet their basic needs—i.e., food and medical supplies (Montesclaros & Caballero-Anthony, 2020). This also applies to gig workers, who faced a reduction in demand for their services (e.g., riding apps). Unlike formal employees, they do not receive company benefits such as income support. A survey by the AppJobs Institute shows that only 23% of these workers have money saved, and that close to 70% of them had no income and were dissatisfied with the support provided by their companies (Moulds, 2020).

### *Access to Commodities*

These effects can be worsened by the impacts of lockdowns on domestic access to essential commodities, such as food. When the overcapacity in transport modes leads to a reduction in the amount of food being transported, it could lead to instances of food shortage. Some countries, in fact, have started to restrict their own exports of food. Vietnam, for instance, had restricted its exports of rice for the entirety of April 2020 (Vu, 2020). In April, Russia and Kazakhstan decided to restrict exports of rice, sunseeds, rye, and buckwheat until June 2020, while Cambodia announced plans to ban rice exports, and India stopped signing new rice export contracts as well (de La Hamaide & Trompiz, 2020). This can exacerbate pre-existing vulnerabilities to food- and economic-insecurity, especially for women with fewer job opportunities, and those who are less educated (Centre for Non-Traditional Security Studies, 2020).

## *Housing*

Apart from this, another risk factor for the lower income group is housing. Whether it be poorer individuals, or workers who migrate overseas for work, it is likely that some of them will be unable to afford housing and other facilities where proper social distancing can be practiced. In Singapore, for instance, one of the key challenges was the ballooning number of COVID-19 cases in foreign worker dormitories. In spite of Singapore's limitations with regards to physical space, the government nonetheless worked to compensate by converting properties into community facilities to house foreign workers during the pandemic, and also deploying over 3,000 public officers to support operators of dormitories as well as employees (Cher, 2020; Zhuo, 2020).

## *Risk of Disorder and Potential Virus Resurgence*

When poorer individuals cannot find formal work opportunities to adapt to the crisis, or when their skillsets do not match the available jobs, they may have to look for alternative work opportunities in informal markets, even if these imply disobeying the lockdown policies. In the worst case scenarios, when even such informal opportunities are not available, they may turn to the streets and engage in protests to demand for more support (Centre for Non-Traditional Security Studies, 2020). Protests have already occurred in multiple countries such as Lebanon, France, and Italy (Mroue, 2020).

The problem with protests is that while they are normally signs of healthy democracies, their occurrence at this time effectively negate whatever gains that were received from previous quarantine policies.

It even puts to waste previous government investments in wage and income support (to be discussed in the next section), and could lead to a resurgence of the virus. In the United States, for instance, anti-lockdown demonstrators/protesters have travelled "hundreds of miles, returning to all parts of their states" based on their mobile phone data (Wilson, 2020, para. 1), making them potential vectors of COVID-19. Therefore, if the economic crisis is uncontrolled, it could have negative implications on the health crisis, as it implies a prolonged time period needed for lockdowns— i.e., until the virus transmissions are significantly reduced or eradicated.

## Priorities in Preventing Crises

The extent of economic impacts of COVID-19 will depend on the stances taken by governments in addressing them, and their capacities to enact timely interventions. A number of potential interventions can potentially be leveraged.

### *Domestic Support to Companies*

Earlier, three channels of impact from health crisis were described: (1) the impacts of border closures, (2) the impacts of shutdowns, and (3) their spill-over effects. The first order of the day is that governments may seek to minimise the direct effects of quarantines on the economy, by ensuring that trade and investment channels are kept open.

However, in cases when such losses cannot be feasibly addressed, the priority is to prevent disruptions from spiralling into a crisis. Such measures, as will be described later, have been projected by the ADB (2020a) to provide improvements of USD1.7 trillion to 3.4 trillion in both three- and six-month scenarios, over the current situation.

On the producers' side, companies need to be supported so that they are not forced to lay off workers and/or cut salaries. In Australia, for instance, the government is providing an SME Guarantee Scheme, guaranteeing 50% of new loans made by SMEs (Australian Government Treasury, 2020). A larger share of up to 90% was in fact guaranteed by the Singapore government under the Temporary Bridging Loan Programme, the SME Working Capital Loan programme, and the Enterprise Financing Scheme–Trade Loan scheme (Choo, 2020). These are important because keeping businesses afloat amid the pandemic is key to preventing a worse crisis, with businesses passing the burden to employees and citizens through lay-offs and salary drawdowns.

In the Philippines, the Bureau of Internal Revenue has, in response to requests from business groups, effectively delayed the deadline for filing income taxes (Parcon, 2020). In the case of essential industries as well as logistics industries, governments may provide them with more support such as inspection services and testing of personnel, as announced in Malaysia (Malaysian Investment Development Authority, 2020).

## *Providing Support to Individuals*

Beyond financial support to companies, governments are also supporting citizens by providing them with opportunities to remain productive amid the lockdowns. This has the dual effect of minimising the disruptive impact of the pandemic on consumption behaviour, while also helping to boost their morale. The United States, for instance, is providing a stimulus package of US$1,200 to Americans earning below US$75,000 annual income, and for every child they have, they were given an additional US$500 ("Coronavirus: Trump signs", 2020). Singapore likewise provided a strong fiscal response to COVID-19 in four of its budgets: the main budget ("Unity budget"), as well as three supplementary budgets ("Resilience", "Solidarity", and "Fortitude" budgets), with a total of close to S$100 billion being allocated (Ministry of Finance, 2020). This includes payments according to the sector impacted, with up to 75% of the first S$4,600 of monthly wages paid and an additional S$600 according to the Ministry of Finance (Choo, 2020).

While some may associate consumer support policies with "Universal Basic Income" policies that pay individuals regardless of employment, an important point is the need to optimise the manner of delivering consumer support policies. In particular, these budgets may backfire, if they promote "couch-potato" mentality, such that people choose to stay home rather than work (Cowen & Kasparov, 2020). For instance, S$2 billion was allocated by the Singapore government for the purpose of creating 100,000 new work opportunities for individuals. These include 40,000 new jobs in childhood education, healthcare, healthcare declaration assistants/swabbers, computer engineers, and machine operators; 25,000 traineeships for younger individuals in fast-growing industries such as information technology and engineering, as well as mid-career traineeships (i.e., attachments); and 30,000 highly subsidised skill upgrading programmes (Ministry of Finance, 2020).

## Supporting Countries with Poor Fiscal Health

However, not all countries have the means to intervene as the abovementioned countries have done. This is because such government spending goes beyond the income levels of economies, also known as "deficit spending", and necessitates the need to borrow funds. For economies that are already mired in debt and fiscal deficits, these would need to be paid at a cost based on the prevailing interest rate. According to the IMF, over 33 countries today are at either high risk of debt distress, or are already going through it (IMF, 2020b). Therefore, governments with lower fiscal health will likely be constrained from implementing the needed economic stimulus policies to counter the effects of lockdowns, making them vulnerable to recessions. The international community is providing assistance to some of these countries, through concessional loans by the IMF, as well as fast-track facilities by the World Bank for funding immediate healthcare needs (IMF, 2020b; Shalal, 2020). Such assistances can go a long way in preventing macroeconomic shocks from occurring, as unsustainable levels of debt may lead to debt- and currency-crises (Iwata *et al.*, 2015).

## Safeguarding Supply Chains for Essential Commodities

Another way to minimise the disruptive impact of the crisis is to ensure that supplies of essential commodities are unperturbed. For instance, the Association of Southeast Asian Nations (ASEAN) is committing 10% from their ASEAN Development Fund/cooperation funds with other countries, to support the provision of medical supplies, with further commitment to ensure the reliability of supply chains for essential commodities such as food, and to ensure that trade and investment channels continue to be open (ASEAN, 2020a). There have likewise been joint supply chain agreements signed by ASEAN Ministers on Agriculture and Fishery (AMAF), designed to secure regional food supply chains, and to facilitate the transportation of food and agricultural products (ASEAN, 2020b).

## Re-examining Critical Infrastructure

The notion of critical infrastructure (CI) commonly applies to "systems and assets that are so vital to the United States that their incapacity or destruction would have a debilitating impact on our physical or economic security or public health or safety" (United States Department of Homeland Security, 2019, para. 1). As society approaches a "new normal" where low-probability and high-impact events (also known as "black-swans") in the form of novel pandemics may occur, this definition of CI will need to be expanded. Housing for poorer populations will need to be seriously considered as a type of CI, as spaces where social distancing is not possible can easily become hotspots for incubating future pandemics, which in turn, leads to protracted lockdowns.

Equally important is the need for new thinking on re-engineering the physical spaces where business is done, including travel between and within countries, office set-ups, dining (restaurants and cafes), sports and recreation, and even mass events, among others. These can act as a "weak link" that could deal a significant blow to the economy as well. Beyond physical infrastructure, the softer infrastructure of protocols will need to be re-examined as well, such as how quarantine and social-distancing for citizens who have travelled abroad should be done. From a cultural perspective, disincentives to calling in sick will need to be addressed, as well as the primacy of having a balanced and healthy lifestyle.

## Developing the "Next Generation" Healthcare Capacity

The international community will need to provide as much support as needed in order to speedily develop vaccines for the current pandemic. However, in the face of uncertainty on future novel diseases, more investment will be needed in the capacity to test, monitor, and analyse novel diseases. Currently, China's investments, at US$1.94 billion, have outstripped other countries, which is approximately triple that of the next biggest investor, Japan (US$640 million), as reflected in an Economist Intelligence Unit (EIU) briefing on COVID-19 (Economist Intelligence Unit, 2020).

Healthcare investments will also need to target the most advanced and comprehensive technologies. Compared to existing methods of reverse transcription polymerase chain reaction (RT-PCR) mentioned in the EIU's website, the tools of whole-genome sequencing or next generation genome sequencing tools are more comprehensive. The latter technologies offer a three- to five-week advantage over existing tools, time which can be used by policymakers to call and enforce lockdowns earlier, cutting the odds of the virus reaching the stage where it is in today (as cited in Montesclaros *et al.*, 2018; Montesclaros, 2020).

These may take longer to establish, and will need to be matched with personnel training, in order to raise a "next-generation army" of healthcare workers that specialised in testing, monitoring, and analysing novel diseases to ascertain their source and provide timely and accurate policy advice. A culture of transparent information sharing across governments will also need to be developed (Montesclaros *et al.*, 2018), anchored on the understanding that no country is self-sufficient in protecting the health of its constituents.

## Conclusion: "This Time is Different"

Referring to the 2007–2008 Global Financial Crisis (GFC) as well as previous economic crises, Carmen Reinhart and Kenneth Rogoff famously argued that "no matter how different the latest financial frenzy or crisis always appears, there are usually remarkable similarities with past experience from other countries and from history" (Reinhart & Rogoff, 2009, p. xxv). In the case of today's crisis, the phrase "this time is different" may just be right, and this allows for two potential perspectives moving forward. On the one hand, the negative perspective may say that the global GDP contractions are nothing like anything that has ever been faced in the past, and that this causes society to retrogress by a few years. If it is worse than the GFC, it could mean that the effects of the virus will last for a decade or more.

On the other hand, a silver lining can be seen in terms of the economic impact. Unlike the GFC, no significant amount of wealth has vanished into the hands of imprudent lenders, borrowers, brokers, and company chiefs. Moreover, the debts of companies today are increasing incrementally for every month that they do not operate. This is unlike the GFC when there was a one-time large increase in debt equal to years' worth of savings. The time required for recovery is thus more controllable, and businesses can potentially work with governments to ride out the pandemic, and rely on them for help. During the GFC, some actors were rightly punished for their imprudent behaviour (as in the case of Lehman Brothers), although this spilled-over into businesses in other sectors/countries who took no part in the crime, thus causing recessions. In contrast, today's "Great Lockdown" has resulted from a disruption that was practically unavoidable from a societal standpoint. The other silver lining is thus that today's crisis has drawn government support and international cooperation. If resources continue to be diverted to those who need them most, a recovery that is quicker than the GFC is not impossible. In fact, Nobel Laureates Abhijit Banerjee and Esther Duflo illustrated this with the notion of a "COVID-19 Marshall Plan" that paralleled post-World War II financing for economic recovery (Banerjee & Duflo, 2020).

Hopefully, this experience with a black swan event makes the international community more resilient in the long-term by being better prepared for future potential disruptions. This includes learning to manage information better, re-examining CI security, growing their reserves to prepare for such emergencies, and investing early in developing a next-generation army of healthcare workers. The hope is that the next novel contagious virus remains a virus, and is not given the space to become a pandemic, in turn, avoiding the additional social and economic costs seen today.

## Acknowledgement

I would like to express my gratitude to Professor Mely Caballero-Anthony, Professor of International Relations at the S. Rajaratnam School of International Studies (RSIS), Nanyang Technological University (NTU), Singapore, and Head of the Centre of Non-Traditional Security Studies (NTS Centre), for providing feedback on an earlier draft of this manuscript, and to Professor Jorgen Schlundt of the NTU Food Technology Centre (NAFTEC) and Chair of the 2019 Global Microbial Identifier Meeting in NTU for previous collaborations which shed light on "next-generation genome sequencing" technologies.

## References

Accenture. (2020, March 29). *From survival to revival: Industrial post COVID-19.* https://www.accenture.com/sa-en/insights/industrial/coronavirus-industrial-post-covid19

Asian Development Bank. (2020a). *Updated assessment of the potential economic impact of COVID-19. ADB Brief, No. 133.* https://www.adb.org/publications/updated-assessment-economic-impact-covid-19

Asian Development Bank. (2020b, March 6). *The economic impact of the COVID-19 outbreak on developing Asia.* ADB Brief No. 128, March. https://www.adb.org/sites/default/files/publication/571536/adb-brief-128-economic-impact-covid19-developing-asia.pdf

ASEAN. (2020a, April 14). *Declaration of the Special ASEAN Summit on Coronavirus Disease 2019 (COVID-19).* https://asean.org/storage/2020/04/FINAL-Declaration-of-the-Special-ASEAN-Summit-on-COVID-19.pdf

ASEAN. (2020b, 17 April). *ASEAN pledges to ensure food security during COVID-19 outbreak.* https://asean.org/asean-pledges-ensure-food-security-covid-19-outbreak/

Australian Government Treasury. (2020, 26 May). *Coronavirus SME Guarantee Scheme—supporting the flow of credit.* https://treasury.gov.au/coronavirus/sme-guarantee-scheme

Banerjee, A., & Duflo, E. (2020, 26 May). Abhijit Banerjee and Esther Duflo on how economies can rebound. *The Economist.* https://www.economist.com/by-invitation/2020/05/26/abhijit-banerjee-and-esther-duflo-on-how-economies-can-rebound

Bermingham, F. (2020, February 21). Coronavirus hits China's farms and food supply chain, with further spike in meat prices ahead. *South China Morning Post.* https://www.scmp.com/economy/china-economy/article/3051737/coronavirus-hits-chinas-farms-and-food-supply-chain-further

Centre for Non-Traditional Security Studies. (2020). *World Hunger Day amidst the COVID-19 pandemic: Priorities in preventing food protests.* NTS Bulletin. https://www.rsis.edu.sg/wp-content/uploads/2020/05/NTS-Bulletin-May-2020-.pdf

Cher, A. (2020, April 22). Why Singapore's push to contain coronavirus among migrant workers is so difficult. *CNBC News.* https://www.cnbc.com/2020/04/23/coronavirus-cases-spike-among-singapore-migrant-workers.html

Choo, Y. T. (2020, April 6). Govt to increase risk share on loans to 90 per cent to ensure credit access for firms during Covid-19 crisis: DPM Heng. *The Straits Times.* https://www.straitstimes.com/politics/government-to-increase-risk-share-on-loans-to-90-per-cent-to-ensure-credit-access-for-firms

Coronavirus: Trump signs. (2020, 30 March). *BBC News.* https://www.bbc.com/news/world-us-canada-52070718

Coronavirus pandemic: Which politicians and celebs are affected? (2020, 17 May). *Al Jazeera.* https://www.aljazeera.com/news/2020/03/coronavirus-pandemic-politicians-celebs-affected-200315165416470.html

COVID-19: Impact could cause equivalent of 195 million job losses, says ILO chief. (2020, April 8). *UN News.* https://news.un.org/en/story/2020/04/1061322

Cowen, T., & Kasparov, G. (2020, May 15). Coronavirus is making universal basic income look better, but the U.S. economy has to get more productive to make UBI feasible. *Bloomberg Opinion.* https://www.bloomberg.com/opinion/articles/2020-05-15/coronavirus-is-making-universal-basic-income-look-better

de La Hamaide, S., & Trompiz, G. (2020, April 4). Trade restrictions on food exports due to the coronavirus pandemic. *Reuters.* https://www.reuters.com/article/us-health-coronavirus-trade-food-factbox/trade-restrictions-on-food-exports-due-to-the-coronavirus-pandemic-idUSKBN21L332

Debucquet, D. L., & Martin, W. (2018). Implications of the global growth slowdown for rural poverty. *Agricultural Economics, 49*(3), 325–338. https://doi.org/10.1111/agec.12419

Economist Intelligence Unit (2019). *2019 Global Health Security Index.* https://www.ghsindex.org/

Economist Intelligence Unit (2020, February 17). *Coronavirus: A Special on Infectious Diseases in Asia* [Webinar].

Elliott, L. (2020, 12 March). Prepare for the coronavirus global recession. *The Guardian.* https://www.rsis.edu.sg/rsis-publication/nts/global-health-security-the-burden-of-covid-19-urgent-need-for-social-safety-nets/#.XsKu6Wgzbb0

Gandhi, M., Yokoe, D. S., & Havlir, D. V. (2020). Asymptomatic transmission, the Achilles' heel of current strategies to control COVID-19. *The New England Journal of Medicine, 382*(22), 2158-2160. https://doi.org/10.1056/NEJMe2009758

Govindarajan, V., & Bagla, G. (2020, May 25). As Covid-19 disrupts global supply chains, will companies turn to India? *Harvard Business Review.* https://hbr.org/2020/05/as-covid-19-disrupts-global-supply-chains-will-companies-turn-to-india

International Monetary Fund [IMF]. (2020a, April). *World Economic Outlook, April 2020: The Great Lockdown.* https://www.imf.org/en/Publications/WEO/Issues/2020/04/14/World-E.conomic-Outlook-April-2020-The-Great-Lockdown-49306

International Monetary Fund [IMF]. (2020b). *List of LIC DSAs for PRGT-Eligible Countries.* https://www.imf.org/external/Pubs/ft/dsa/DSAlist.pdf

International Monetary Fund [IMF]. (2020c). https://www.imf.org/en/News/Articles/2020/04/13/pr20151-imf-executive-board-approves-immediate-debt-relief-for-25-countries

Iwata, C., Montesclaros, J. M. L., & Qi, X. (2015). Systemic risks of ASEAN+3 financial integration: Challenges, opportunities and the future. *Revista Digital Mundo Asia Pacífico, 4*(6). https://doi.org/10.17230/map.v4.i6.05

Malaysian Investment Development Authority. (2020, May 21). *Restricted Movement Order (RMO) for Malaysia Industries.* https://www.mida.gov.my/home/restricted-movement-order-(rmo)-for-malaysia-industries/posts/

Ministry of Finance (2020). *Ministerial Statement on Support Measures in Our Continuing Fight Against the Covid-19 Pandemic.* https://www.singaporebudget.gov.sg/docs/default-source/budget_2020/download/pdf/fy2020_fortitude_budget_statement.pdf

Montesclaros, J. M. L., Caballero-Anthony, M., & Schlundt, J. (2018). *Supporting the Genome Microbial Identifier and Whole Genome Sequencing in Addressing Food-Borne Diseases in ASEAN.* https://www.rsis.edu.sg/wp-content/uploads/2018/11/PR181121_Supporting-the-Genome-Microbial-Identifier-and-Whole-Genome.pdf

Montesclaros, J. M. L. (2020, February 20). *Beyond COVID-19: Global Priorities Against Future Contagion.* https://www.rsis.edu.sg/rsis-publication/nts/beyond-covid-19-global-priorities-against-future-contagion/#.XxSgKkBuI2x

Montesclaros, J. M. L., & Caballero-Anthony, M. (2020, March 19). *Global Health Security—The Burden of COVID-19: Urgent Need for Social Safety Nets.* https://www.rsis.edu.sg/rsis-publication/nts/global-health-security-the-burden-of-covid-19-urgent-need-for-social-safety-nets/#.XsLSMGgzbb0

Moulds, J. (2020, April 21). Gig workers among the hardest hit by coronavirus pandemic. *World Economic Forum.* https://www.weforum.org/agenda/2020/04/gig-workers-hardest-hit-coronavirus-pandemic/

Mroue, B. (2020, April 28). Riots in impoverished north Lebanon city amid currency crash. *Associate Press.* https://apnews.com/db74186fbe34f0dc5fac32046e4f5f01#:~:text=BEIRUT%20(AP)%20%E2%80%94%20Clashes%20broke,the%20protests%20turned%20into%20riots

Naftulin, J. (2020, April 7). WHO says there is no need for healthy people to wear face masks, days after the CDC told all Americans to cover their faces. *Business Insider.* https://www.businessinsider.sg/who-no-need-for-healthy-people-to-wear-face-masks-2020-4?r=US&IR=T

Nebehay, S. (2020, February 3). WHO chief says widespread travel bans not needed to beat China virus. *Reuters.* https://www.reuters.com/article/us-china-health-who/who-chief-says-widespread-travel-bans-not-needed-to-beat-china-virus-idUSKBN1ZX1H3

Parcon, J. A. (2020). *A reprieve from tax filing during COVID-19.* PwC Philippines. https://www.pwc.com/ph/en/taxwise-or-otherwise/2020/a-reprive-from-tax-filing-during-covid-19.html

Quah, E., & Swee, E. (2020, June 18). Lives v livelihoods debate—The economist's take. *The Straits Times.* https://www.straitstimes.com/opinion/lives-v-livelihoods-debate-the-economists-take

Reinhart, C. M., & Rogoff, K. S. (2009). *This time is different: Eight centuries of financial folly.* Princeton University Press.

Shalal, A. (2020, March 28). World Bank, IMF urge debt relief for poorer countries hit by coronavirus. *Reuters.* https://www.reuters.com/article/us-health-coronavirus-world-bank-relief/world-bank-imf-urge-debt-relief-for-poorer-countries-hit-by-coronavirus-idUSKBN21E2O9

UNESCAP. (2012). *Policy Guidebook for SME Development in Asia and the Pacific.* https://www.unescap.org/resources/policy-guidebook-sme-development-asia-and-pacific

United States Department of Homeland Security (2019, October 23). *Critical Infrastructure Security.* https://www.dhs.gov/topic/critical-infrastructure-security#:~:text=Critical%20infrastructure%20describes%20the%20physical,or%20public%20health%20or%20safety

Vos, R., Martin, W., & Laborde, D. (2020, March 10). *As COVID-19 spreads, no major concern for global food security yet.* International Food Policy Research Institute Blog. https://www.ifpri.org/blog/covid-19-spreads-no-major-concern-global-food-security-yet

Vu, K. (2020, April 28). Vietnam PM says to fully resume rice exports from May. *Reuters.* https://www.reuters.com/article/us-vietnam-rice-exports/vietnam-pm-says-to-fully-resume-rice-exports-from-may-idUSKCN22A1SN

WHO. (2010, February 24). *What is a pandemic?* https://www.who.int/csr/disease/swineflu/frequently_asked_questions/pandemic/en/

WHO. (2020a, February 16). *Coronavirus disease 2019 (COVID-19) Situation Report.* https://www.who.int/docs/default-source/coronaviruse/situation-reports/20200216-sitrep-27-covid-19.pdf?sfvrsn=78c0eb78_4

WHO. (2020b, March 11). *WHO Director-General's opening remarks at the media briefing on COVID-19.* https://www.who.int/dg/speeches/detail/who-director-general-s-opening-remarks-at-the-media-briefing-on-covid-19---11-march-2020

WHO. (2020c, March 19). *Considerations for quarantine of individuals in the context of containment for coronavirus disease (COVID-19).* https://www.who.int/publications/i/item/considerations-for-quarantine-of-individuals-in-the-context-of-containment-for-coronavirus-disease-(covid-19)

Wilson, J. (2020, May 18). US lockdown protests may have spread virus widely, cellphone data suggests. *The Guardian.* https://www.theguardian.com/us-news/2020/may/18/lockdown-protests-spread-coronavirus-cellphone-data

Worldometer. (2020). *COVID-19 Coronavirus Pandemic.* https://www.worldometers.info/about/

Xu, M., Zhang, S., & Kumar, D. K. (2020, February 14). Stranded tankers, full storage tanks: Coronavirus leads to crude glut in China. *Reuters.* https://www.reuters.com/article/us-china-health-oil-storage/stranded-tankers-full-storage-tanks-coronavirus-leads-to-crude-glut-in-china-idUSKBN2072NR

Zhuo, T. (2020, May 28). Singapore ambassador to US rebuts Foreign Policy article on Covid-19 outbreak in dorms. *The Straits Times.* https://www.straitstimes.com/singapore/singapore-ambassador-to-united-states-rebuts-foreign-policy-article-on-covid-19-outbreak

Chapter 3

# Enhancing Collective Community Resilience Throughout a Pandemic: Insights from Singapore

Pamela Goh

## Introduction

The world witnessed the massive outbreak of the novel coronavirus (2019-nCoV) in late 2019; it became commonly known as COVID-19 and was declared a pandemic by March 2020. Fear and anxiety are common responses during a health crisis (Lin, 2020), as people inevitably and naturally worry for their own well-being. The change of Singapore's Disease Outbreak Response System Condition (DORSCON) level from the yellow to orange category had resulted in the self-serving and panic-driven rush of Singaporeans to purchase and stock up on various groceries, household items (Tan, 2020), and other important items such as surgical masks (Chia, 2020), leaving little to no stocks for others.

When the circuit breaker measure was implemented by the local government, most workplaces were closed and moved online, except for essential services such as clinics and restaurants; schools similarly proceeded to home-based online learning as well (Abu Baker, 2020a). Additionally, Singaporeans speedily took action to reduce their susceptibility to the virus by engaging in greater levels of hygiene practices (e.g., regularly washing hands), avoiding crowded places, and not travelling to other countries (Ho, 2020). Among many other countries in the world, Singapore also imposed travel restrictions for China for an indefinite period of time. Despite this implemented measure, some Singaporeans started an online petition to ban the entry of Chinese nationals into Singapore (Smith, 2020). Indeed, the COVID-19 pandemic has led to the manifestation of xenophobic and racial sentiments in the online sphere, which may cause fractures and disruption to Singapore's social harmony.

Singapore rushed to contain the spread of the pandemic as the number of local cases escalated exponentially, with new clusters forming in both the community and among the migrant worker dormitories (Kok, 2020). Nonetheless, while the government may establish and implement however many strict measures in response to COVID-19, these measures can only do so much to combat the spread of the coronavirus. Complementing these government initiatives is also the need for the community to both agree with and actually engage in the various coping initiatives. Indeed, collective action is necessary for successful management of the pandemic, highlighting the need to build resilience in residents and ultimately across the society as a whole. In this endeavour to build community resilience that will undoubtedly contribute to the country's overall efforts to sustain itself during the crisis, community leaders have an indispensable role to play, serving as important figures that the various communities in Singapore can turn to for guidance. In this chapter, four key strategies will be shared on what individuals and community leaders can do during a pandemic, to help in the containment of the health crisis.

## Strategy #1: Emphasise Personal Responsibility in the Continuous Combat Against the Spread of the Pandemic

In health pandemics, the first line of defence in combatting and containing the crisis lies with individuals. Raising awareness about the importance of personal responsibility in combatting the pandemic is necessary to prompt the proactive, actual manifestation of such behaviours in individuals. For instance, this can be done by informing the public on some of the consequences of falling ill as a result of the coronavirus. A potential concern that may arise is that doing so could lead to unnecessary panic and anxiety in the community, and this must be balanced by neither over-stating nor over-emphasising the detrimental consequences of falling ill. Nonetheless, it remains that such initiatives may help the public recognise how real the threat is and what they can do, which in turn is likely to encourage them to take the initiative to enhance self-protection. COVID-19 has shown signs of persisting as another endemic virus, with no clear signs of cessation in the near future (Tham, 2020). In other words, individual health behaviours need to continue, even if the coronavirus should show signs of containment in the community.

Different people have different levels of risk tolerance and require different levels of need for safety. Some people may downplay the risks of and their susceptibility to the coronavirus, whereas others may perceive a stronger need to take additional precautions, engaging in their respective hygiene practices that they believe in and are comforted by. Ultimately, the degree of effort that individuals undertake to protect themselves from the crisis should be respected. Nonetheless, entrusting the community to contribute to the overall crisis response efforts during the pandemic is a reflection of empowerment bestowed upon the community. Individuals are trusted to be capable and know what to do to protect themselves (Leonard, 2019) against the coronavirus, without excessive government intervention.

Community leaders and individuals themselves can serve as role models for the public, by following guidelines on what they should or should not do to protect themselves in the face of the pandemic. It is also important to highlight how real the threat of the pandemic is by informing the public on the detrimental consequences of falling ill to the coronavirus. For instance, the community can be informed that there is still no known cure for the coronavirus (Wee, 2020), and that the virus is highly contagious with real cases of human-to-human transmission (Lovelace, 2020). The public is always in the best position to protect themselves, and part of this includes encouraging people to change maladaptive practices and, more importantly, continuing to engage in adaptive ones. Social responsibility is repetitively emphasised, and Singaporeans are always encouraged to avoid becoming complacent. Even with the stabilisation of viral spread and reduction in community infection—thereby promoting the recommencement of social activities and businesses to a certain degree upon the lifting of the circuit breaker—people in Singapore are still encouraged to adhere to social distancing rules and to minimise social gatherings wherever possible (Abu Baker, 2020b; Lim, 2020).

Ultimately, external initiatives as such have limited effect, unless people proactively and consistently undertake these behaviours to help themselves. The individual efforts of residents will contribute to a collective effect of community resilience against the health crisis.

# Strategy #2: Engage in Consistent and Effective Crisis Communications to Address Questions, Fears, and Uncertainty

## *Provide Information to Keep the Community Updated on Crisis Developments*

The continuous and prompt dissemination of both health advisories and updates on the health pandemic is critical in allaying public fear and anxiety. By keeping the community up-to-date on developments and the various concrete ways in which they can enhance their protection against the virus, a sense of psychological safety can be fostered. An important outcome of this initiative is the minimisation of negative emotional reactions in the community, such as fear (Hess, 2017). For instance, the new measure undertaken by the government to provide free surgical masks to each household (Khalik & Goh, 2020), which eventually progressed to the giving out of cloth masks to each resident (Yang, 2020), serves to contain social anxiety through reassurances that there are sufficient masks for everyone. Additionally, the continuous process of providing information to the community helps to foster trust in leaders because it conveys the message that the leaders are on top of things, and the public will not be kept in the dark with regards to any crisis information or development. In turn, the public is likely to turn to community leaders as authentic and reliable information providers. Since the emergence of the first infected individual in Singapore, the government has held regular press conferences to address and explain the developments in the pandemic. This included informing the public on matters relating to infected cases, to the rationale behind varying government measures targeted at tackling the coronavirus, and even what the community can and should expect with regards to the health crisis.

Sharing important information and addressing any concerns/questions of the public is critical in keeping the community updated. While information is imparted to the public, details need to be similar to and consistent with official sources of information. This is vital to prevent confusion in the midst of anxiety. During the pandemic, however, crisis communications can be severely restricted, making it difficult for community leaders to physically reach out to the residents. Community leaders have to be mindful and thus creative in the manner through which they deliver information to the wider public. Alternative methods have to be considered, such as online tools like Facebook videos that can help to reach out to the wider community instantly and easily. More importantly, leaders also have to ensure that their alternative methods of delivering information are appropriate and tailored for the different demographic groups in the community. This may include the poor who may not be able to afford the internet and thus do not have access to social media, or the elderly who may not be well-versed in online modes of communication.

Health advisories are also a means of delivering important information to the public. Hence, the dissemination of such informative materials should continue. These materials should educate people on the right hygiene etiquette that they should engage in, as well as other critical facts necessary to keep them sufficiently informed about the crisis. Such advisories could also serve as a platform to debunk myths by providing "do you know" information, including the explanations behind these myths and truths. Health advisories could also serve to provide vital contact details that the community can reach out to for further help, including mental healthcare hotlines. In Singapore, the National CARE hotline was established with the specific purpose of helping anyone who require emotional assistance. In an attempt to reach out to the different demographic groups in the community through these advisories, these materials should similarly be tailored according to needs, such as the language used and communication style.

## *Combat Fake News Swiftly*

The health crisis can, unfortunately, be exploited to further induce public panic, through the spread of fake news. For instance, information that a person in Singapore, who was infected with the virus, had passed away was inaccurately shared and spread in the online HardwareZone Forum ("POFMA Office", 2020); this piece of fake news was quickly addressed by the authorities. Thus, the act of intervening in the spread of fake news can prevent further fear and anxiety emerging in the public.

The provision of information in a timely and transparent manner is necessary to foster trust in news sources (Kuck *et al.*, 2009). When there is trust by the community in these legitimate news sources, such as official health advisories from the Ministry of Health, people would be less inclined to turn to alternative and potentially inaccurate sources of information. In turn, the spread of fake news can be minimised. Even if fake news were to successfully emerge and spread, the public would likely seek to confirm these details against the information published on authentic and official news platforms.

Efforts to detect and debunk any fake news should include the swift provision, sharing, and dissemination of accurate information in response to fake news. Alternatively, the community could be directed to official news platforms to obtain their information regarding the pandemic. Concurrently, it is vital to remind the community not to share any unverified information, even if it is done out of goodwill—i.e., to warn others because it is "better to be safe than sorry". In the same vein, considerations must be made to ensure that the different demographic groups in the community are also being educated on the presence of fake news during a pandemic. Similar communication channels utilised for providing the community with developments in the health crisis can also be used for debunking fake news.

## Strategy #3: Rally the Community Together in the Face of the Pandemic

The presence of xenophobic and racial sentiments in Singapore can fuel hatred towards certain members of society, and disrupt Singapore's existing social harmony. When the public is rallied together in times of a crisis, it helps to create a collective identity among the people (Rao, 2018), which in turn will lead to more supportive and empathetic behaviour towards each other.

### *Engage in Dialogues with the Community*

Having conversations with members of the community would help leaders understand the sentiments and concerns that are brewing on the ground. When issues surface, leaders can address them promptly, thus preventing the escalation of these issues. This includes addressing any misconceptions that the public might have, as surfaced and identified in conversations. Social tensions in the community could hence be avoided in the midst of the health crisis, which would subsequently reduce anger, hatred, and social disharmony.

Regular ground-sensing initiatives allow for community leaders to understand the community's thoughts and feelings towards the pandemic. When the community's concerns are heard and misconceptions are addressed, they can better cope with the health crisis. Opportunities to engage with the public could be done either by opening formal communication platforms for the public to turn to, or for leaders to informally walk the ground and interact with the community. Vulnerable populations should be heard as well, such as the elderly and poor, to ensure that all stakeholder voices are respected.

Engaging in dialogues with the community can be difficult during a health crisis where social distancing measures are put in place to combat the spread of the virus. Other methods of reaching out to the community have to be employed, the most common of which is social media. Leaders in Singapore have taken to Facebook to reach out to residents during the COVID-19 pandemic. Upon the lifting of the circuit breaker measure, leaders immediately returned to the ground to interact with the residents, continuing to wear masks, and maintaining a safe distance with others while setting a good example for the local community.

## Encourage People to Stand United and React Rationally to the Crisis

The act of standing together in times of crisis is necessary to promote societal harmony, wherein people will come together and support each other in solidarity and empathy (Goh & Neo, 2020). When people are reminded that everyone is experiencing the crisis, it emphasises that everyone has a stake in the crisis regardless of their background or country of origin. The outcome is that a sense of unity redirects people's focus from putting the blame on specific groups of people for the cause and spread of the coronavirus towards engaging in active efforts to combat the health pandemic together.

Being empathetic and supportive of one another helps to unite the community in solidarity in times of a crisis as such. As imperative as it is to appeal to the community to be rational and not act solely on their emotions in reaction to the crisis, it is also vital to remind people to respect each other's practices and beliefs. Before the pandemic escalated in Singapore and everyone was required to wear a mask when they are outside, for instance, this could be in the form of not shunning those who still chose to wear one despite feeling well and not having the need to. With the implementation of the circuit breaker, it became mandatory for everyone to wear a mask whenever they were outside in public; if not, they run the risk of being fined (Yong, 2020b). In such circumstances, acts of support could simply come in the form of reminders to one another, to bring and wear a mask when needed and whenever outside of one's residence.

In response to the COVID-19 pandemic in Singapore, the SG United movement (SG UNITED, 2020) was established to rally citizens together. The initiative allows Singaporeans to come together to help one another in the face of the health crisis, through various means such as volunteering or donating to the needy through various organic campaigns. People were also collectively involved in showing appreciation for the front liners by clapping their hands and singing songs from the windows of their homes during the circuit breaker period ("Sing along to Home", 2020).

## Strategy #4: Strive to Achieve Normalcy, or Even the New "Norm", During a Pandemic

The need to maintain normalcy is also vital in times of adversity (Lin *et al.*, 2009). While it is important for people to be kept up to date with the progress of COVID-19, it is concurrently essential that people do not become preoccupied with news reports of the crisis. Doing so may increase the likelihood of further anxiety and an unhealthy obsession with engaging in protective actions, which ultimately can disrupt the community's ability to function on a day-to-day basis.

Efforts to limit the spread of the virus have been undertaken to protect the community; schools and organisations are encouraged to undertake precautionary measures to protect students and staff. When the community is informed and reassured that they are being looked after, it prompts trust in community leaders and thus government. In other words, it helps to not excessively draw away people's attention and resources onto the health pandemic, but instead allows people to return to their daily routine. Subsequently, as people regain a sense of control of their lives, feelings of panic and anxiety should reduce.

The public should also be highly encouraged to continue their normal way of life despite the disruptions and measures, while looking out for one another if possible. This includes remaining calm and not engaging in potentially selfish behaviours, such as panic buying. Volunteering to help with the various vulnerable communities in the society, or simply educating them, is also a way to help such groups retain a certain degree of functioning during a pandemic.

As the pandemic progresses towards stabilisation and containment, certain measures have to continue to be put in place as the country looks into reopening its economy. Absolute return to how the country was performing prior to the pandemic is impossible; after all, the usual daily routines have to take into account precautionary measures in order to contain the spread of the virus (Yong, 2020a). A sense of uncertainty will persist and adjustments have to be recalibrated constantly depending on the continuing development of the health crisis. Adaptation to these new changes may be wearing and stressful, but is still necessary in order to resume a certain degree of daily functioning once more.

## Conclusion

Building community resilience during a health pandemic contributes to the recovery efforts in response to the crisis. There are various ways to build community resilience, such as endorsing the importance of personal responsibility in the continuous combat of the pandemic, engaging in consistent and effective crisis communications, rallying citizens together, and even striving to achieve normalcy or the new "norm". When the community comes together, people will respond with hope and positivity in the face of a crisis—even in a pandemic with an uncertain prognosis, it could potentially and eventually be contained and managed.

## Acknowledgement

The views expressed in this chapter are the author's only and do not represent the official position or view of the Ministry of Home Affairs, Singapore.

## References

Abu Baker, J. (2020a, June 2). Singapore's circuit breaker and beyond: Timeline of the COVID-19 reality. *Channel News Asia.* https://www.channelnewsasia.com/news/singapore/covid-19-circuit-breaker-chronicles-charting-evolution-12779048

Abu Baker, J. (2020b, June 4). Real risk of resurgence in COVID-19 cases, clusters if too many activities resume too quickly: Gan Kim Yong. *Channel News Asia.* https://www.channelnewsasia.com/news/singapore/real-risk-resurgence-covid19-reopen-too-quickly-gan-kim-yong-12802586

Chia, R. G. (2020, January 30). These 12 Twitter posts show the insane queues for masks in Singapore, Shanghai and Hong Kong, which are all sold out. *Business Insider.* https://www.businessinsider.sg/photos-and-videos-show-insane-queues-for-masks-in-singapore-shanghai-and-hong-kong-which-netizens-say-are-all-sold-out/

Goh, P., & Neo, L. S. (2020). *Stronger than before: 6 lessons from the Surabaya bombings.* Singapore, Home Team Behavioural Sciences Centre.

Hess, E. (2017, January 17). Here's why emotions are the secret sauce of innovation. *Forbes.* https://www.forbes.com/sites/darden/2017/01/17/the-secret-sauce-of-innovation-emotions/#4a630fa57116

Ho, K. (2020, January 29). Three in five of Singaporeans afraid of contracting the Wuhan coronavirus. *YouGov.* https://sg.yougov.com/en-sg/news/2020/01/29/three-five-singaporeans-afraid-contracting-wuhan-c/

Khalik, S., & Goh, T. (2020, January 31). Wuhan virus: Each Singapore household to get 4 free masks for contingencies. *The Straits Times.* https://www.straitstimes.com/singapore/health/each-spore-household-to-get-4-free-masks-for-contingencies

Kok, X. (2020, April 28). Coronavirus: Singapore's Covid-19 cases to rise as not all migrant workers are being tested. *South China Morning Post.* https://www.scmp.com/week-asia/health-environment/article/3078199/coronavirus-singapore-100-1000-infections-one-month

Kuck, X., Lin, L. A., Tan, A., Khader, M., & Ang, J. (2009). *Managing community resilience during the Influenza A (H1N1) virus threat* (Research Report No. 11/2009). Singapore: Home Team Behavioural Sciences Centre.

Leonard, K. (2019, February 9). What are the benefits of employee empowerment? *Chron.* https://smallbusiness.chron.com/benefits-employee-empowerment-1177.html

Lim, M. Z. (2020, June 15). Phase 2 of Singapore's reopening: What you can do from June 19. *The Straits Times.* https://www.straitstimes.com/singapore/what-you-can-do-from-june-19-when-singapore-goes-into-phase-2-of-reopening

Lin, S. (2020, January 29). Commentary: SARS was scary, but the experience was invaluable in shaping our Wuhan virus response. *Channel News Asia.* https://www.channelnewsasia.com/news/commentary/wuhan-virus-singapore-cases-response-sars-2003-quarantine-12360244

Lovelace, B. J. (2020, February 4). Researchers say the coronavirus may be more contagious than current data shows. *Consumer News and Business Channel.* https://www.cnbc.com/2020/02/04/researchers-say-the-coronavirus-may-be-more-contagious-than-current-data-shows.html

Ministry of Health. (2020). *Advisories for various sectors.* https://www.moh.gov. sg/2019-ncov-wuhan/advisories-for-various-sectors

POFMA Office issues correction notice to SPH Magazines over HardwareZone Forum post on Wuhan virus. (2020, January 27). *Channel News Asia.* https:// www.channelnewsasia.com/news/wuhan-virus-moh-gan-kim-yong-instructs-pofma-issue-correction-12352752

Rao, S. (2018, July 30). The term "Asian American" was meant to create a collective identity. What does that mean in 2018? *The Washington Post.* https:// www.washingtonpost.com/lifestyle/style/the-term-asian-american-was-meant-to-create-a-collective-identity-is-it-necessary-in-2018/2018/07/27/c30e7eb0-8e90-11e8-b769-e3fff17f0689_story.html

SG United. (2020). https://www.sgunited.gov.sg

Sing along to Home on April 25 to express thanks to frontline and migrant workers. (2020, April 24). *Today.* https://www.todayonline.com/singapore/sing-along-home-april-25-express-thanks-frontline-and-migrant-workers-0

Smith, L. M. (2020, January 28). Wuhan virus: Over 100,000 sign online petition calling for Singapore to ban travelers from China. *Business Insider Singapore.* https://www.businessinsider.sg/wuhan-virus-over-100000-sign-online-petition-calling-for-singapore-to-ban-travellers-from-china/

Tan, A. (2020, February 8). Coronavirus: Politicians, supermarkets urge calm amid panic-buying of groceries. *The Straits Times.* https://www.straitstimes. com/singapore/health/coronavirus-fairprice-chief-urges-calm-amid-panic-buying-of-groceries-singapores

Tham, Y-C. (2020, May 15). Covid-19 could be here to stay: WHO expert. *The Straits Times.* https://www.straitstimes.com/world/covid-19-could-be-here-to-stay-who-expert

Wee, S-L. (2020, February 5). In coronavirus, China weighs benefits of buffalo horn and other remedies. *The New York Times.* https://www.nytimes. com/2020/02/05/world/asia/coronavirus-traditional-chinese-medicine.html

World Health Organization. (2020). *Novel Coronavirus (2019-nCoV).* https:// www.who.int/emergencies/diseases/novel-coronavirus-2019

Yang, C. (2020, May 7). Coronavirus: New cloth masks for all residents as Singapore ramps up production. *The Straits Times.* https://www.straitstimes. com/singapore/health/new-cloth-masks-for-all-residents-as-spore-ramps-up-production

Yong, M. (2020b, April 15). COVID-19: What the law says about having to wear a mask when outside your home. *Channel News Asia.* https://www. channelnewsasia.com/news/singapore/covid-19-singapore-masks-going-out-law-12643120

Yong, C. (2020a, May 21). Coronavirus: People will have to get used to new normal, says PM Lee. *The Straits Times.* https://www.straitstimes.com/singapore/people-will-have-to-get-used-to-new-normal-says-pm-lee

# Chapter 4

# Mitigating the Social Pandemic of Xenophobia During COVID-19

Nur Aisyah Abdul Rahman

## Introduction

As the COVID-19 virus spread to various countries around the world, there were also reports of virus-related prejudice. There have been many reported cases of discrimination towards Chinese and Chinese-looking people around the world since the virus was determined to have originated from Wuhan, China (Yan *et al.*, 2020). In one incident in Los Angeles, a man verbally abused a Thai American man in public and claimed "Every disease has ever came from China" (Yan *et al.*, 2020, para 11). In March 2020, a Singaporean student in London was physically assaulted by a group of local youths. One of the attackers said to him, "I don't want your coronavirus in my country" (Yong, 2020, para 6). Closer to home, there were reports of people shunning Chinese nationals and businesses (Lee & Loke, 2020).

The impact of such prejudice extended to the other communities in Singapore. Abdul Halim Abdul Karim, an Islamic religious teacher in Singapore, claimed in a Facebook post that the COVID-19 outbreak was retribution for China's oppressive treatment of Chinese Muslim Uighurs (Kurohi, 2020). Even after being investigated by the authorities and issuing a public apology, his incendiary comments continued to anger many netizens. For some netizens, Abdul Halim's claims were an attack

55

on people of Chinese ethnicities and non-Muslims in general. Some people were not satisfied with his apology and brought up past instances of communal tensions where Muslims were targeted. One netizen commented, "Said sorry and move on? The Melayu [Malay] community was not so forgiving when Chinese do the same thing to them, why now Chinese must be forgiving when Malays were not? Hypocrisy much?" (Abdul Rahman, 2020).

In April 2020, the outbreak of infection clusters among the migrant worker population living in dormitories led to a drastic surge in the number of cases (Badalge, 2020). As of May 2020, there were over 33,000 cases in total—from about 1,000 cases in March—with the migrant worker population making up the majority of recent infections (Ministry of Health, 2020). The surge in cases shifted the xenophobic focus from Chinese nationals to the migrant worker populations, most of whom are from Bangladesh, India, and China (Sin, 2020). For example, there was a Whatsapp message being widely circulated that claimed these migrant workers were infecting foreign domestic workers, and thus infecting their Singaporean employers and families (Sin, 2020).

These incidents show that pandemics such as COVID-19 can stir up social tensions. In such times, policymakers need to pay attention to not only the medical effects of the virus, but also the social effects that can spill over into the long run. By using the Integrated Threat Theory[1] (Stephan & Stephan, 2000), this chapter will explore how the COVID-19 outbreak has exacerbated xenophobia, and suggest strategies to address these issues.

## How has COVID-19 Exacerbated Xenophobia?

According to the Integrated Threat Theory, prejudice towards an outgroup (i.e., people of a different social group than one's own) can arise from realistic and symbolic threats to the ingroup (i.e., people of the same social group; Stephan & Stephan, 2000).

---

[1] The Integrated Threat Theory (ITT) or intergroup threat theory is a social psychology theory has often been used to explain intergroup conflict, including various forms of prejudice (e.g., Islamophobia, right-wing extremism, racism, homophobia). ITT assumes that people innately categorise themselves based on shared characteristics and relate the group's well-being to their own.

## *Realistic Threats*

Realistic threats are factors that threaten the existence of the ingroup or the physical well-being of its members. These include loss of resources, threats to physical safety, threats to the ingroup's power, and psychological and economic threats—e.g., crime, disease, limited economic opportunities, unemployment (Ciftci, 2012; Stephan & Stephan, 2000).

According to the evolutionary psychology perspective, humans have evolved to detect parasites, pathogens, and diseases that can harm themselves or their ingroup survival (Schaller & Neuberg, 2012). For example, have you ever moved away or caught yourself feeling disgusted by someone with eczema, even when you knew it is not a contagious skin condition? Or, perhaps you reflexively shot a dirty look at someone who coughed in the train recently? The "behavioural immune system" enables humans to identify cues of the disease quickly (e.g., physical disfigurements, coughing), and elicit avoidance behaviours to ensure one's protection (Huang *et al.*, 2011; Schaller & Neuberg, 2012).

However, this disease-avoidance mechanism is not perfect. It might even cause a false positive and lead people to avoid others with non-contagious illnesses. Research has found that people who are more sensitive to diseases are more likely to show avoidant behaviours and attitudes towards people with non-contagious health conditions (e.g., people with disabilities or obesity), especially when a threat of infection is made salient (Schaller & Neuberg, 2012). This disease-avoidance mechanism can be generalised to all perceived outgroup members (Cottrell & Neuberg, 2005). With news of the "novel coronavirus threat from China" or the "Wuhan virus" dominating mass media, there is a constant implicit association of the virus with the race of potential carriers. Hence, contributing to prejudice against specific races.

Even among ingroup members, group boundaries might be altered. There is a risk of victims of COVID-19 to be stigmatised by their social network, including their own families. COVID-19 is still a relatively unknown virus. The lack of information on such emerging threats can amplify the fear of infection and encourage discrimination. Unlike obvious physical threats such as terror attacks, biological threats are invisible to the naked eye and can be deeply frightening (Center of Study of Traumatic Stress, 2001). These uncertainties can lead to irrational fears of prolonged periods of infection, causing victims and their families to be stigmatised and isolated in the long run. Surveys of victims of the SARS epidemic and their family in Hong Kong and China revealed that victims felt stigmatised, while some family members reported being embarrassed to be part of a SARS-afflicted family (Tsang *et al.*, 2004). In Singapore, there are also reports of discrimination that has extended to frontline healthcare workers, with nurses in uniform being verbally abused and forced out of public transportation (Lay, 2020), as well as an ambulance driver who was denied food service for fear of infection (Tan, 2020).

All these fears in times of crisis can compound and exacerbate existing points of tension. In Singapore, issues of immigration, especially relating to foreign talent employees and students, have been a salient faultline in the past few decades (Mathews *et al.*, 2019). Foreigners are perceived to be displacing locals and competition for economic and educational opportunities. The migrant worker population is also stereotypically linked with crime. In a poll by the International Labour Organisation (2019), 52% of Singaporean respondents held the view that an increase in crime rates could be attributed to migrant workers. The threat of infectious disease, compounded with existing tension, can thus embolden people to lash out in defence of their ingroup.

## Symbolic Threats

Symbolic threats emerge when the ingroup perceives that an outgroup is trying to undermine the ingroup's worldview with their own (Stephan & Stephan, 2000). Groups' worldviews are expressed through their ingroup identity, values, customs, religions, national identity, and traditions. Perceived violation of ingroup identity and values can lead to prejudice and negative sentiments towards outgroup members (Ciftci, 2012).

Some people have attributed the virus outbreak to poor personal hygiene habits and exotic cultural diets (e.g., eating dogs and bats). The COVID-19 virus was traced to a wet market in Wuhan, where wildlife meat was sold (Woodward, 2020). Around the same time, videos of Asians eating bats and other exotic wildlife, allegedly in Wuhan, were gaining attention online, with netizens claiming that these were the origins of the outbreak (Sadler, 2020). One of these videos featured a woman named Wang Mengyun eating bat soup at a restaurant. In an interview, Wang revealed that the video she was in was part of a 2016 travel programme shot in Micronesia (Sadler, 2020). The footage had been taken out of context, and sensationalised by netizens and media outlets alike (Ramirez, 2020), thus further stoking xenophobic and racist sentiments.

Even though the majority of Singaporean citizens are ethnically Chinese, Singaporean Chinese perceive themselves to be culturally different from Chinese nationals (Jacobs, 2012; Yeoh & Lin, 2013). In Singapore, incidents such as the notorious Ferrari car crash[2] and presumably Chinese migrants defecating or allowing their children to defecate in public spaces have led to outrage targeted at Chinese nationals in particular (Loh, 2015; Stolarchuk, 2018; Yeoh & Lin, 2013). As infection clusters appeared within the migrant worker population in April 2020, a forum letter was published in the Chinese daily newspaper, Lianhe Zaobao. The writer, linked the COVID-19 outbreak among migrant workers to the workers' unhygienic practices, minimising the fact that their cramped living space is a factor in accelerating the spread of the virus (Lee, 2020). In this light, Chinese nationals and other migrant workers have been stereotyped to possess conflicting values and incompatible habits (e.g., unhygienic) with the rest of Singaporean society. Prior to the COVID-19 outbreak, Mathews *et al.* (2019) also found that 67.5% of Singaporeans surveyed felt that immigrants, in general, are not doing enough to integrate. A substantial proportion of participants also expressed discomfort with having immigrants as family members (Mathews *et al.*, 2019). Given such pre-existing tensions and negative sentiments towards immigrants, one can only imagine how easy it is for people to attribute the cause of the virus to the perception of "unadaptable and unhygienic" immigrants.

## What Can We Do to Mitigate the Effects?

Clearly, resolving prejudice and discrimination in society is no easy feat. Its insidious and deep-rooted nature makes it difficult for researchers and policymakers to identify a single magic bullet. Yet, if left unchecked, prejudice and discrimination can lead to devastating long-term effects

---

[2] In May 2012, an affluent businessman from China who was working in Singapore was involved in a fatal car accident that killed multiple people, including himself. Videos of him running a red light at an intersection and crashing into a taxi went viral, and triggered anti-Chinese national vitriol (Jacobs, 2012).

in social cohesion and resilience. Thus, this section suggests recommendations specific to the COVID-19 situation that may help alleviate the expression of prejudice and discrimination in our society.

## Keeping the Public Informed on COVID-19 Developments Through Public Education

Lacking knowledge on an emerging disease, fear of infection, and existing prejudice can understandably lead to stigmatisation of perceived and actual carriers. It is hence essential that the public is kept informed on recent developments of the COVID-19 situation through public education campaigns. In one study that looked at the stigmatisation of Acquired Immune Deficiency Syndrome (AIDS) and SARS, public education campaigns helped to mitigate stigmatisation in the public (Des Jarlais *et al.*, 2006). These campaigns kept the public updated with transparent and accurate information, such as the incidence of infections during laboratory accidents. With emerging infectious diseases like AIDS and SARS, it took time and education to reduce stigmatisation.

Similarly, the Singaporean authorities have been lauded for keeping the public informed on the developments of the COVID-19 situation (Flam, 2020). For example, there are daily updates on the number of cases, locations that COVID-19 cases have visited, updates on how the virus is transmitted and possible infection prevention methods. Such information is accessible through official websites and news outlets, as well as the Gov.SG channels on WhatsApp and Telegram. The authorities were also prompt to address any misinformation arising from controversial incidents, such as with Abdul Halim and Li Shiwan (Kurohi, 2020; Lim, 2020). This is an effective way of managing misinformation and reducing panic as the situation develops, and thus reducing stigmatisation towards specific communities.

However, it is evident that there are still anxieties about the spread of the virus. Education efforts might need to continue beyond the current crisis period in order to prevent anxieties from creating widespread panic, prolonging, or sparking community tensions. Moreover, the recent shift in the epicentre of the disease is a strong indication that COVID-19 cannot be attributed to any race, culture, or nationality. Emphasising that the infection is not based on race, religion, or nationality, but of proximity, is important in reducing misinformation and stigmatisation. Educating people on how the disease spreads and how they can continue to protect themselves can be useful in the long run to contain the spread of the disease and community tensions.

## *Encouraging Shared Identities and Values*

Another way to reduce the perception of outgroup symbolic threat is to focus on what people might have in common. Gaertner *et al.* (1989) suggest that people have many social identities that fall into three levels: subordinate (i.e., personal identity), basic (i.e., social identity), and superordinate (meta social group identity or human identity).

By focusing on commonalities, people are more likely to perceive others to share the same basic social identity and be part of the same ingroup. Instead of focusing on differences between communities and attributing the cause of the crisis to these differences, there could be more focus on what we have in common. This would encourage people to perceive others to be part of the same ingroup as them. During the current COVID-19 crisis, leveraging on people's religious and national identities might mitigate the socially divisive effects of the outbreak. For example, religious leaders can emphasise religious teachings that encourage compassion and altruism towards those affected by the virus. At the same time, policymakers can focus on the national values of solidarity and brotherhood (i.e., reinforcing the meta social group identity of being Singaporean). In one of his ministerial broadcasts on the COVID-19 situation, Prime Minister Lee highlighted the efforts of volunteers and frontline workers in helping others during the pandemic. He reiterated how "these acts of solidarity and human kindness exemplify the best in us" to rally Singaporeans together (CNA, 2020).

By leveraging on common identities and shared values, more people might be encouraged to be compassionate towards others. Community leaders can encourage ground-up efforts that aid people who are directly affected by the virus. For example, some volunteers have been sending food to quarantined families in Singapore (Wong, 2020). In contrast to some people's xenophobic sentiments, there were also many others involved in ground-up initiatives of compassion directed at migrant workers. Many non-government organisations, charities, businesses, and individuals have coordinated efforts to send migrant workers food, masks, daily supplies, messages of support, and care packages (Ang, 2020; Siswandjo, 2020).

## Encouraging Healthy Social Norms as Part of Community Resilience

Social norms determine what the desirable and acceptable behaviour within a society are (Tankard & Paluck, 2016). It can also signify group membership and identity. In this sense, social norms play a critical role in the discrimination of outgroup members (Schlueter *et al.*, 2013). In times of uncertainty, there might be people who try to take advantage of the situation to elicit division. With people blaming specific communities for the virus, it is important that community leaders encourage healthy social norms, such as compassion and solidarity, to build community resilience. As in the case of Abdul Halim, MUIS representatives had emphasised the teachings of Islam as a peaceful and compassionate religion (Kurohi, 2020). Other local religious teachers also spoke up against the vitriol, calling for unity in this time of crisis. One such person is Mohamad Ghouse Khan Surattee who said on Facebook:

> Now is not the time to blame anyone, or to look it as a punishment or retribution to a specific nation or race... Now the virus is already outside our doorstep, blaming the outbreak (on others) at this moment could delay the valuable help.

Promptly denouncing divisive sentiments and encouraging shared values are integral to rallying people together. Reinforcing ground-up acts of compassion, such as sending food to families under quarantine (Wong, 2020), and sharing of protective medical supplies (e.g., hand sanitiser, masks; Cheng & Mohan, 2020), serves to emphasise a sense of community and solidarity of the community.

Considering that health pandemics bring about repercussions for social cohesion, community resilience movement as part of the pandemic response can mitigate the negative impact of these issues. SGUnited is a national initiative launched by the Ministry of Culture, Community and Youth (MCCY) to specifically safeguard Singapore's resilience and cohesion in the face of the COVID-19 crisis. The SGUnited website echoes messages of resilience and unity, features stories of compassion and altruism, provides resources for people to get help, and provides a platform for individuals to get involved and coordinate volunteer efforts. While campaigns, such as SGUnited, might start as top-down efforts, using them as a medium to promote ground-up efforts, effectively provides a recognisable label to these helping behaviours. This label reflects healthy social norms of solidarity, compassion, and resilience in the face of crisis. In the event of another national crisis in the future, reusing such labels can encourage similar resilient behaviours and embed it into the national identity.

## Acknowledgement

The views expressed in this chapter are the author's only and do not represent the official position or view of the Ministry of Home Affairs, Singapore.

## References

Abdul Rahman, N. A. (2020). *COVID-19: A biological and social pandemic?* (HTBSC research report 14/2020). Singapore: Home Team Behavioural Sciences Centre.

Ang, P. (2020, April 19). Coronavirus: We will look after you, ministry assures foreign workers. *The Straits Times.* https://www.straitstimes.com/singapore/we-will-look-after-you-ministry-assures-foreign-workers

Badalge, K. N. (2020, April 22). Surge in coronavirus cases in Singapore forces lockdown extension. *Al Jazeera.* https://www.aljazeera.com/news/2020/04/surge-coronavirus-cases-singapore-forces-lockdown-extension-200422060-906200.html

Center of Study of Traumatic Stress. (2001). *Planning for bioterrorism: Behavioral and mental health responses of weapons of mass destruction and mass disruption.* http://www.dtic.mil/dtic/tr/fulltext/u2/a392688.pdf

Cheng, I., & Mohan, M. (2020, February 6). "The kampung spirit is still alive": Punggol residents step up amid coronavirus outbreak. *CNA.* https://www.channelnewsasia.com/news/singapore/wuhan-coronavirus-singapore-virus-punggol-kampung-spirit-12397614

Ciftci, S. (2012). Islamophobia and threat perceptions: Explaining anti-Muslim sentiment in the West. *Journal of Muslim Minority Affairs, 32*(3), 293–309. https://doi.org/10.1080/13602004.2012.727291

CNA. (2020, June 7). *PM Lee Hsien Loong on Singapore's post-COVID-19 future, says "Do not fear" | National broadcast* [Video]. YouTube. https://www.youtube.com/watch?v=rAhuD368Ij0

Cottrell, C. A., & Neuberg, S. L. (2005). Different emotional reactions to different groups: A sociofunctional threat-based approach to "prejudice". *Journal of Personality and Social Psychology, 88*(5), 770–789. https://doi.org/10.1037/0022-3514.88.5.770

Des Jarlais, D. C., Galea, S., Tracy, M., Tross, S., & Vlahov, D. (2006). Stigmatisation of newly emerging infectious diseases: AIDS and SARS. *American Journal of Public Health, 96*(3), 561–567. https://doi.org/10.2105/AJPH.2004.054742

Flam, F. (2020, March 1). Singapore's coronavirus transparency has lessons for the U.S. *Bloomberg Opinion.* https://www.bloomberg.com/opinion/articles/2020-03-01/trump-coronavirus-plan-should-take-a-page-from-singapore

Gaertner, S. L., Mann, J., Murrell, A., & Dovidio, J. F. (1989). Reducing intergroup bias: The benefits of recategorisation. *Journal of Personality and Social Psychology, 57*(2), 239–249. https://doi.org/10.1037/0022-3514.57.2.239

Huang, J. Y., Sedlovskaya, A., Ackerman, J. M., & Bargh, J. A. (2011). Immunising against prejudice: Effects of disease protection on attitudes toward outgroups. *Psychological Science, 22*(12), 1,550–1,556. https://doi.org/10.1177/0956797611417261

International Labour Organization (2019). *Public attitudes towards migrant workers in Japan, Malaysia, Singapore, and Thailand.* https://www.ilo.org/wcmsp5/groups/public/---asia/---ro-bangkok/documents/publication/wcms_732443.pdf

Jacobs, A. (2012, 26 July). In Singapore, vitriol against Chinese newcomers. *The New York Times.* https://www.nytimes.com/2012/07/27/world/asia/in-singapore-vitriol-against-newcomers-from-mainland-china.html

Kurohi, R. (2020, February 8). MHA, Muis investigating religious teacher's posts. *The Straits Times.* https://www.straitstimes.com/singapore/mha-muis-investigating-religious-teachers-posts

Lay, B. (2020, February 8). Anecdotes online claim S'pore nurses ostracised for taking MRT in uniform & spreading viruses. *Mothership.* https://mothership.sg/2020/02/nurses-mrt-uniform-wuhan-virus/

Lee, J. (2020, April 15). Covid-19 outbreak in dorms due to migrant workers' poor hygiene & bad habits: Zaobao forum letter. *Mothership.* https://mothership.sg/2020/04/migrant-workers-zaobao-letter/

Lee, M., & Loke, L. (2020, February 19). Some Chinese workers, businesses in Singapore shunned amid fear and anxiety over Covid-19. *Today.* https://www.todayonline.com/singapore/some-chinese-workers-businesses-singapore-shunned-amid-fear-and-anxiety-over-covid-19

Lim, Y. L. (2020, April 18). Coronavirus: Letter on dorm cases xenophobic, says Shanmugam. *The Straits Times.* https://www.straitstimes.com/singapore/letter-on-dorm-cases-xenophobic-shanmugam

Loh, A. (2015, October 20). Woman relieves herself besides train station, public shocked. *The Online Citizen.* https://www.theonlinecitizen.com/2014/08/14/woman-relieves-herself-besides-train-station-public-shocked/

Mathews, M., Lim, L., & Selvarajan, S. (2019). IPS-ONEPEOPLE.SG indicators of racial and religious harmony: Comparing results from 2018 and 2013.

*Institute of Policy Studies*. https://lkyspp.nus.edu.sg/docs/default-source/ips/ips-working-paper-no-35_ips-onepeoplesg-indicators-of-racial-and-religious-harmony_comparing-results-from-2018-and-2013.pdf

Ministry of Health. (2020, May 28). *Daily report on COVID-19*. https://www.moh.gov.sg/docs/librariesprovider5/2019-ncov/situation-report---28-may-2020.pdf

Ramirez, M. N. (2020, February 27). Coronavirus: How Fox News and other right-wing media endanger our health. *USA Today*. https://www.usatoday.com/story/opinion/2020/02/27/fox-news-right-wing-media-conspiracy-theories-coronavirus-COVID-19-column/4886082002/

Sadler, R. (2020, January 28). Coronavirus: "Racism" behind people blaming woman eating bat soup for virus. *Newshub*. https://www.newshub.co.nz/home/world/2020/01/coronavirus-racism-behind-people-blaming-woman-eating-bat-soup-for-virus.html

Schaller, M., & Neuberg, S. (2012). Danger, disease, and the nature of prejudice(s). *Advances in Experimental Social Psychology, 46*, 1–54. https://doi.org/10.1016/B978-0-12-394281-4.00001-5

Schlueter, E., Meuleman, B., & Davidov, E. (2013). Immigrant integration policies and perceived group threat: A multilevel study of 27 Western and Eastern European countries. *Social Science Research, 42*(3), 670–682. https://doi.org/10.1016/j.ssresearch.2012.12.001

Sin, Y. (2020, April 30). Covid-19 outbreak brings migrant workers from margin to centre of Singapore's attention. *The Straits Times*. https://www.straitstimes.com/opinion/migrant-workers-from-margin-to-centre-of-spores-attention

Siswandjo, P. (2020, March 2). Local volunteer groups show care and concern to foreign workers amidst COVID-19. *The Pride*. https://pride.kindness.sg/local-volunteer-groups-show-care-and-concern-to-foreign-workers-amidst-covid-19/?utm_source=FB&utm_medium=FB-CTW&utm_campaign=SDL_SKM_02_03_20_local_volunteer_groups_show_care_concern_foreign_workers_amidst_covid_19&utm_content=local_volunteer_groups_show_care_concern_foreign_workers_amidst_covid_19&fbclid=IwAR0dBPq2FJWIvuZvbT7UvGuC8uy_o9lSh8A7fLQ_1utwVDjwdhLsLjCoR5Y

Stephan, W., & Stephan, C. W. (2000). An integrated threat theory of prejudice. In S. Oskamp (Ed.), *Reducing Prejudice and Discrimination* (pp. 23–46). Lawrence Erlbaum Associates Publishers.

Stolarchuk, J. (2018, October 5). "This is normal in China!"—Woman who brings her grandson to poop in public lashes out at Singaporeans. *The Independent*. http://theindependent.sg/this-is-normal-in-china-woman-who-brings-her-grandson-to-poop-in-public-lashes-out-at-singaporeans/

Tan, A. (2020, February 8). S'pore ambulance driver allegedly turned away from food stall, according to Grab driver. *Mothership*. https://mothership.sg/2020/02/grab-driver-story-of-ambulance-driver/

Tankard, M. E., & Paluck, E. L. (2016). Norm perception as a vehicle for social change. *Social Issues and Policy Review, 10*(1), 181–211. https://doi.org/10.1111/sipr.12022

Tsang, H. W. H., Scudds, R. J., & Chan, E. Y. L. (2004). Psychosocial impact of SARS. *Emerging Infectious Diseases, 10*(7), 1,326–1,3277. https://doi.org/10.3201/eid1007.040090

Wong, P. T. (2020, February 14). Faceless "Santa Clauses" make grocery runs for family observing home quarantine. *Today.* https://www.todayonline.com/singapore/faceless-santa-clauses-make-grocery-runs-family-observing-home-quarantine

Woodward, A. (2020, February 27). Both the new coronavirus and SARS outbreaks likely started in Chinese wet markets. Photos show what the markets look like. *Business Insider.* https://www.businessinsider.sg/wuhan-coronavirus-chinese-wet-market-photos-2020-1?r=US&IR=T

Yan, H., Chen, N., & Naresh, D. (2020, February 21). What's spreading faster than coronavirus in the US? Racist assaults and ignorant attacks against Asians. *CNN.* https://edition.cnn.com/2020/02/20/us/coronavirus-racist-attacks-against-asian-americans/index.html

Yeoh, B. S. A., & Lin, W. (2013). Chinese migration to Singapore: Discourses and discontents in a globalising nation-state. *Asian and Pacific Migration Journal, 22*(1), 31–54. https://doi.org/10.1177%2F011719681302200103

Yong, C. (2020, March 5). UK police release images of 4 men linked to COVID-19 racist attack on Singaporean student in London. *The Straits Times.* https://www.straitstimes.com/singapore/uk-police-release-images-of-4-men-linked-to-COVID-19-racism-attack-on-singaporean-student

# Section 2

# Psychological Well-Being
# Related Issues

# Chapter 5

# How to Cope with Mental Health Issues During a Pandemic

Cherie Chan and Adrian Toh

## Introduction

Imprints of psychosocial impact were observed in each of the 21st century pandemics that the world's populations endured. Varying degrees of psychological effects such as anxiety (often reported as distress, fear, panic, and worry), anger, depression, insomnia, social isolation, loneliness, post-traumatic stress, and stigmatisation were reported across different pandemics (Coughlin, 2012; Jalloh *et al.*, 2018; Röhr *et al.*, 2020; Tsang *et al.*, 2004; Zheng *et al.*, 2005).

It would be surprising if psychosocial responses to COVID-19 differed. In fact, at the time of this writing, preliminary findings from local surveys have revealed increased mental health concerns and reports of family violence during the COVID-19 period (Tai, 2020). While the primary focus during a pandemic is on the vigilance and fight against the infectious disease, the psychosocial aspect is as important. With the lack of timely and effective care, the compromised psychosocial aspect may consequently lead to increased vulnerability to mental health issues, decreased ability to cope and function occupationally and interpersonally. This chapter will focus on ways to cope with mental health issues during a pandemic, based on lessons learnt in this and past pandemics, so as to be better prepared to respond in the future.

## Keeping Things in Perspective

The amount of information regarding the COVID-19 situation in Singapore and the world can be overwhelming. Notably, the confusion and uncertainty about the virus, the potential threat and the loss of situational awareness may heighten anxiety, stirring up feelings of fear and anger. While it is natural for one to seek out information to gain a better understanding of the situation to influence one's locus of control (the belief of control over the situations and experiences that affects one's life), it is important to seek out information that is reflective of the situation (as opposed to misinformation).

During the COVID-19 outbreak in Singapore, there was misinformation (fake news and rumours) circulating among the public. The content included advice not to visit certain public hospitals, death of individuals due to the infection, to avoid a list of places where suspected or confirmed cases had been, and claims by Prime Minister Lee that he was tested positive (Ministry of Health, 2020b). These items were circulated through mediums such as text messaging services (e.g., WhatsApp) and social media (e.g., Facebook). The intent of circulating fake news may stem from the perception that the news is real or, alternatively, from the perception that it is a harmless joke to share such information. However, the impact of the circulation of fake news is detrimental. It affects the individual's emotions, such as fostering an increased sense of fear (e.g., of being infected, the lack of household essentials), and potentially leading to changes in the individual's behaviours (e.g., panic-buying).

Consequently, these behaviours disrupt the management of the pandemic situation in Singapore (e.g., leading to a short-term shortage of supplies, increased queueing and congregation). Our brains are wired to respond to threats and dangers in the environment, an evolutionary imprint inherited for survival function. When faced with severe threats, neural activity is increased in the amygdala, an area of the brain that processes strong emotions such as fear (Morelli *et al.*, 2020). During such times, increased activity in the amygdala may overpower the frontal lobes, which guides thinking, reasoning, decision-making and planning. Consequently, behaviours are driven by fight-or-flight responses, which explains the above-mentioned behaviours.

As a result, communication with the right authority becomes even more critical in enhancing mental health outcomes. A study by Lin *et al.* (2018)

found that a combination of interpersonal communication with health networks and intrapersonal factors such as concern about health and knowledge about how viruses are transmitted, determined the adoption of non-pharmaceutical interventions (NPI) and vaccines. This suggests that communication of information by the right professionals and authority figures could help with overall adoption of pro-social behaviour, which then leads to better mental health outcomes. The sharing of information today can be widespread within a short duration of time. While there can be attempts to minimise such spread by the authorities, individuals can also take an active role in managing and communicating information as it appears on our mobile devices. Below are some steps that we can take to manage better when we receive distressing information:

1. Stay calm, notice your breathing.
2. Notice current triggered emotions.
3. Consider the source of information.
4. Re-read the content of the information with a curious mind.
5. Observe the content in light of the current understanding.
6. Evaluate the content critically.
7. Consider the consequences of circulation.
8. If the information is evaluated as misinformation, play a part to discourage the circulation.

## Building Resilience

The COVID-19 situation has significant implications on health, emotional, and social functioning, with the need to address uncertain prognosis, severe shortages, and large financial losses as part of the bigger pandemic response (Pfefferbaum & North, 2020). Singapore was not spared when COVID-19 hit hard in February 2020; it led to a variety of emotions and reactions. Many individuals hoarded items such as masks, hand sanitisers, and alcohol wipes. For some individuals, this seemed like a normal and necessary action to keep themselves safe and protected. For others, it was deemed unnecessary and shameful. Are these extreme outcomes due to differences in individual resilience?

Resilience is a common buzzword used during pandemics. Huey and Palaganas (2020) shared a list of definitions with a general theme of being able to recover from setbacks and problems effectively, and adapt during adversity. These definitions go beyond just keeping a positive mindset. Resilience has been shown to have a positive impact on mental health and adjustment (An *et al.*, 2016; Hartley, 2011). Building resilience could be the key to helping us choose which of the following pathways to walk on:

1.  Give up and feel like nothing can change, or,
2.  Accept what you cannot change (e.g., a pandemic) and focus on what you can (e.g., how you want to live through this pandemic).

Building resilience involves recovering from and adapting to the environment to better suit one's needs. This could help move one from giving up to focusing on what could be done. This could include:

1.  Keeping yourself connected with others. Having a sense of connection allows you to feel less alone and fearful when facing uncertain situations.
2.  Find ways to be accountable for your actions. Starting a fun project or hobby and inviting friends/family to come on board with these projects could be a common topic for conversations and shared experiences.
3.  Use this situation as a learning experience. As COVID-19 becomes an experience, there might be another time in your life where a pandemic comes up again. Use the current situation to create memories and experiences for use in future conversations and actions.
4.  Switch up and change your environment. Living in a space that brings negativity can lead to feelings of helplessness and pain. Bringing in plants, using music and creating a more relaxed ambience could be helpful in creating a more purposeful space to just be in.

When individuals adapt and hold their thoughts and feelings kindly during this pandemic situation, individual resilience is built up with an increased likelihood of coping better with the pandemic.

## Improved Coping With Stress

Apart from the stress and anxieties related to COVID-19, there were other emotional stressors that resulted from the impact of COVID-19, such as being home for a prolonged period due to the "circuit breaker" measure

(Ministry of Health, 2020a). In this section, we will be addressing some of the commonly identified stressors and exploring ways to cope with them.

One of the commonly identified concerns was the stress brought on by working from home (WFH). WFH is not a new phenomenon (some call it telecommuting), and it has been regarded to be a convenient mode of alternative work arrangement. However, not everyone is familiar with such work arrangements, and there are several disadvantages identified by research, such as the lack of social connection, decreased self-esteem, and loneliness (Harpaz, 2002). Also, WFH can result in overworking and burnout. Some strategies that can be useful for individuals who are WFH include the following:

1. Setting specific work goals for the particular day or week.
2. Rewarding self (e.g., a short break) when you reach certain milestones through the day.
3. Being accountable with someone about goals and plans—this can also keep us connected socially.
4. Having clear work boundaries—this includes work hours and physical boundaries (i.e., working in a designated place at home).
5. Having clear and open communication with colleagues or superiors regarding expectations.

Social support is key to many, more so for individuals with mental health concerns. Social support can take many forms, such as meeting up to have a heart-to-heart talk with a close friend over a meal, going hiking or enjoying a picnic by the beach with peers. These activities can help an individual to better manage their emotional difficulties. However, with the implementation of safety measures such as social distancing, it limited the availability of these social resources that many rely on to cope. That said, there are many alternative ways to connect with ourselves and others. With the difficulties brought about by COVID-19, embracing individual factors such as being in touch with our personal feelings could help increase our mental health resiliency and coping. Being able to "A.C.E." your emotions through:

- *A*cknowledging your emotions.
- *C*oming back to your body (labelling where the emotions are in your physical body).
- *E*ngaging your senses to be in the present moment helps ground oneself during such times.

In relation to connecting with others, some of these can include having video calls, playing online group games, or even ordering food for one another and enjoying the food together through video calls. Tsai *et al.* (2010) found that the use of teleconferencing helped alleviate loneliness and depressive symptoms for elderly residents of a nursing home, whose everyday circumstances are similar to and reflective of the circuit breaker that kept everyone in. Teleconferencing tools and video calls could be helpful ways of keeping people connected and maintaining meaningful relationships. Furthermore, being creative and flexible can improve people's mental ability to adapt when the situation changes. Life is full of changes, and some of these changes cannot be controlled. The ability to think flexibly and adapt will help one to revise plans in the face of obstacles, setbacks, new information, or mistakes. Consequently, this will also help them to cope better with the perceived stress.

Another way to cope with stress is to exercise. Exercise has been known to increase one's sense of well-being and overall health. Specifically, in a pandemic situation, exercising brings two major benefits: (1) to cope better with stress, and (2) to improve sleep. These are two protective factors that share a bi-directional relationship. When we exercise, our body releases chemicals called endorphins, which function as the body's natural painkillers and mood elevators (Leuenberger, 2006). At the same time, exercise also reduces the levels of stress hormones, such as adrenaline and cortisol, within the body. Thus, the direct changes to the brain chemistry as a result of exercising can enhance the management of negative emotions during the pandemic situation.

Sleep can be affected by various factors during a pandemic, such as stress experienced throughout the day or a lack of structured routine. Consequently, the lack of sleep can increase vulnerability to many diseases, including infection (Ganz, 2012). Studies (e.g., Driver & Taylor, 2000; Singh *et al.*, 1997) have demonstrated that exercising improves sleep quality and increases sleep duration. With improved sleep, not only does it have a positive effect on stress management, it also relates to having better interpersonal functioning and behavioural coping (Killgore *et al.*, 2008), which would reduce the impact of stress.

## Communication and Compassion

When the circuit breaker started on 7 April 2020, Singapore became a "still city". Food establishments, entertainment venues, retail outlets, and certain healthcare services were brought to a standstill. Telecommuting was the new way of life with delivery and take-aways the only option for "dining out" in what was once a bustling food nation. With this change, individuals reacted in a myriad of ways. Whilst most people abided by circuit breaker rules, some others displayed poor adherence. Individuals even risked fines and became aggressive to bring a sense of normalcy back into their lives. During a pandemic, choices that we make and the manner with which we communicate them can impact our mental health and vice versa.

The combination of effective communication and engagement with social support systems through uncertain times correlates with our ability to cope and participate meaningfully, which can buffer stress, poor mental health, and performance (Kessler *et al.*, 1985). The use of assertive communication plays a key role in coping with the above stated mental health fallouts. As pandemics bring fear and uncertainty, many times our expressed emotions and communication patterns become unhealthy as our minds get caught up with managing perceived or real threats to our survival. Poor interpersonal communication has been found to be a risk factor for mental health (Segrin, 2015), and it would be imperative to keep communication open and assertive to help increase engagement with others around us. For example, practising openness to disagreements, and working on our ability to state our needs clearly would help in de-escalating stress when we engage with another person in a tense situation. Showing compassion and kindness to self when difficult feelings come up instead of engaging in harsh and critical blaming narratives could also contribute to higher levels of positive affect, which leads to better communication and stronger adoption of health-promoting behaviour (Sirois *et al.*, 2015).

Effective communication styles can also lead to increased empowerment within the communities. Empowering individuals through compassion and understanding instead of hard-handed rules can lead to long term partnerships, collaborations, and co-learning, which serve to protect against mental health problems (Nelson *et al.*, 2001; Thompson *et al.*, 2017). In support of this, helping individuals feel empowered through altruism or doing good for others has a significant impact on an individual's decision making. These shifts help move one from a self-interest perspective to one that focuses on optimising resources for the community. This has led to a reduction in costs and mortality, and increases one's self-esteem and usefulness in current times (Shim *et al.*, 2012).

Taken together, compassion and ability to communicate effectively play a significant role in our ability to make choices around connecting with, contributing to, and caring for each other, which then leads to better mental health coping during these uncertain times.

## Caring for Children

As the adults' attention focuses on precautionary measures to protect their families and ensure their safety (e.g., practising good hygiene, avoidance of public places), it is necessary to also consider the psychological well-being of the children in the midst of the pandemic. Children, too, experience substantial changes in their lives due to the pandemic. This would include disruption to their daily routines such as attending school and enrichment classes, socialising at the playground, and birthday celebrations. Research informs that children as young as two years old are aware of changes around them (Stein *et al.*, 2019), and they are well attuned to adults' emotional states. Thus, the exposure to unexplained and unpredictable behaviour by the adults around them may be perceived by children as a threat, resulting in a state of anxiety (Dalton *et al.*, 2020). In fact, in a survey conducted with students (from grades 2 to 6) who were confined at home in Hubei, China, 22.6% reported having depressive symptoms, and 18.9% reported having anxiety symptoms (Xie *et al.*, 2020).

Children may experience and express stress differently in response to the changes, and their responses to stress are easily ignored or misinterpreted. Some behaviours to be watchful for include:

- Returning to behaviours they have outgrown (e.g., bedwetting).
- Being easily irritable or angered.
- Having excessive crying.
- Experiencing unexplained headaches and body aches.
- Having unhealthy eating and/or sleeping habits.
- Having excessive worry or sadness.

To help children to cope, it would be useful for adults to set aside space (which includes time, environment, and emotional space) to speak to the children regarding their concerns and help them make sense of the current situation. Specifically, adults should:

- Normalise their concern, letting them know that it is okay to feel in a particular way.

- Share with them facts in the manner that they can understand, and dispel any false beliefs that they may have. The use of social stories can be useful when communicating with children.
- Provide them with assurance about their (and your) safety—e.g., taking the necessary precautions and looking after one another.
- Discuss with them how you deal with your own stress so that they can model after you (or use some of the tips suggested previously).
- Where possible, limit the child's exposure to news coverage of the event, particularly social media, as children can easily misinterpret information and be frightened about what they do not understand.

## Conclusion

As discussed in this chapter, the impact of COVID-19 goes far beyond economic problems and will likely continue beyond the end of the pandemic. COVID-19 has led to us living in a new era with a "new normal" to grapple with, such as more flexible arrangements in working and living in the future, which also bring its own levels of distress. The mental health fallout from COVID-19 spreads far beyond those who have been infected with the disease. The resulting closures of entertainment and dining establishments, restriction of social gatherings, and cancellations or digitalisation of weddings, funerals, and graduation ceremonies have led to increased stress during a stressful and unpredictable time. Although the impact might be far-reaching, it is important to come back to skills that can help us manage from the inside out. Taking care of ourselves through connecting flexibly and openly with our needs will help us to keep things in perspective and cope better with stressors that are pushed to us through our media channels. Connecting and communicating effectively with our family and loved ones could lead to stronger social units, which in turn contribute to the recovery and resilience of our nation's fight against the virus.

The pandemic situation is ever-evolving, and uncertainty is at its peak. Enhancing the mental well-being of Singaporeans from our frontline staff to our children and the wider community is therefore critical in continuing this battle against new viruses and diseases that may arise. It is imperative to take time to ground ourselves in facts, maintain safe boundaries, and allow ourselves space to make mistakes as we navigate new ground as one nation.

# References

An, H. J., Bae, Y. J., Cho, M. S., Kim, E. H., Kim, Y. O., Lee, Y. L., & Kim, J. (2016). The influence of communication, resilience, mental health on military adjustment of soldiers in the Rear Air Force. *Journal of the Korea Academia-Industrial Cooperation Society, 17*(7), 694–703. https://doi.org/10.5762/KAIS.2016.17.7.694

Coughlin, S. S. (2012). Anxiety and depression: linkages with viral diseases. *Public Health Reviews, 34*(2), 7. https://doi.org/10.1007/BF03391675

Dalton, L., Rapa, E., & Stein, A. (2020). Protecting the psychological health of children through effective communication about COVID-19. *The Lancet Child & Adolescent Health, 4*(5), 346–347. https://doi.org/10.1016/S2352-4642(20)30097-3

Driver, H. S., & Taylor, S. R. (2000). Exercise and sleep. *Sleep Medicine Reviews, 4*(4), 387–402. https://doi.org/10.1053/smrv.2000.0110

Ganz, F. D. (2012). Sleep and immune function. *Critical Care Nurse, 32*(2), e19–e25. https://doi.org/10.4037/ccn2012689

Harpaz, I. (2002), Advantages and disadvantages of telecommuting for the individual, organisation and society. *Work Study, 51*(2), 74–80. https://doi.org/10.1108/00438020210418791

Hartley, M. T. (2011). Examining the relationships between resilience, mental health, and academic persistence in undergraduate college students. *Journal of American College Health, 59*(7), 596–604. https://doi.org/10.1080/07448481.2010.515632

Huey, C. W. T., & Palaganas, J. C. (2020). What are the factors affecting resilience in health professionals? A synthesis of systematic reviews. *Medical Teacher*, 1–11. https://doi.org/10.1080/0142159X.2020.1714020

Jalloh, M. F., Li, W., Bunnell, R. E., Ethier, K. A., O'Leary, A., Hageman, K. M., Sengeh, P., Jalloh, M. B., Morgan, O., Hersey, S., Marston, B. J., Dafae, F., & Redd, J. T. (2018). Impact of Ebola experiences and risk perceptions on mental health in Sierra Leone. *BMJ Global Health, 3*(2), http://dx.doi.org/10.1136/bmjgh-2017-000471

Kessler, R. C., Price, R. H., & Wortman, C. B. (1985). Social factors in psychopathology: Stress, social support, and coping processes. *Annual Review of Psychology, 36*(1), 531–572. https://doi.org/10.1146/annurev.ps.36.020185.002531

Killgore, W. D., Kahn-Greene, E. T., Lipizzi, E. L., Newman, R. A., Kamimori, G. H., & Balkin, T. J. (2008). Sleep deprivation reduces perceived emotional intelligence and constructive thinking skills. *Sleep Medicine, 9*(5), 517–526. https://doi.org/10.1016/j.sleep.2007.07.003

Leuenberger, A. (2006). Endorphins, exercise, and addictions: a review of exercise dependence. *The Premier Journal for Undergraduate Publications in the Neurosciences, 3*, 1–9.

Lin, L., McCloud, R. F., Jung, M., & Viswanath, K. (2018). Facing a health threat in a complex information environment: A national representative survey examining American adults' behavioral responses to the 2009/2010 A (H1N1) pandemic. *Health Education & Behavior*, *45*(1), 77–89. https://doi.org/ 10.1177/1090198117708011

Ministry of Health, Singapore (2020a). *Circuit breaker to minimise further spread of COVID-19*. https://www.moh.gov.sg/news-highlights/details/ circuit-breaker-to-minimise-further-spread-of-covid-19

Ministry of Health, Singapore (2020b). *Clarifications on misinformation regarding COVID-19*. https://www.moh.gov.sg/covid-19/clarifications.

Morelli, N., Rota, E., Immovilli, P., Spallazzi, M., Colombi, D., Guidetti, D., & Michieletti, E. (2020). The Hidden Face of Fear in the COVID-19 Era: The Amygdala Hijack. *European Neurology*, 1.

Nelson, G., Lord, J., & Ochocka, J. (2001). Empowerment and mental health in community: narratives of psychiatric consumer/survivors. *Journal of Community and Applied Social Psychology*, *11*(2), 125–142. https://doi. org/10.1002/casp.619

Pfefferbaum, B., & North, C. S. (2020). Mental health and the Covid-19 pandemic. *New England Journal of Medicine*. https://doi.org/10.1056/ NEJMp2008017

Röhr, S., Müller, F., Jung, F., Apfelbacher, C., Seidler, A., & Riedel-Heller, S. G. (2020). Psychosocial impact of quarantine measures during serious coronavirus outbreaks: A rapid review. *Psychiatrische Praxis*, *47*(4), 179–189. https://doi.org/10.1055/a-1159-5562

Segrin, C. (2015). Communication and mental health. *The International Encyclopedia of Interpersonal Communication*, 1-5. https://doi.org/10.1002/ 9781118540190.wbeic012

Shim, E., Chapman, G. B., Townsend, J. P., & Galvani, A. P. (2012). The influence of altruism on influenza vaccination decisions. *Journal of The Royal Society Interface*, *9*(74), 2,234–2,243. https://doi.org/10.1098/rsif. 2012.0115

Singh, N. A., Clements, K. M., & Fiatarone, M. A. (1997). A randomised controlled trial of the effect of exercise on sleep. *Sleep*, *20*(2), 95–101. https://doi.org/10.1093/sleep/20.2.95

Sirois, F. M., Kitner, R., & Hirsch, J. K. (2015). Self-compassion, affect, and health-promoting behaviors. *Health Psychology*, *34*(6), 661. https://doi. org/10.1037/hea0000158

Stein, A., Dalton, L., Rapa, E., Bluebond-Langner, M., Hanington, L., Stein, K. F., Ziebland, S., Rochat, T., Harrop, E., Kelly, B., & Bland, R. (2019). Communication with children and adolescents about the diagnosis of their own life-threatening condition. *The Lancet*, *393*(10176), 1,150–1,163. https://doi.org/10.1016/S0140-6736(18)33201-X

Tai, J. (2020, May 8). Mental health fallout: How Covid-19 has affected those in Singapore. *The Straits Times*. https://www.straitstimes.com/singapore/health/mental-health-fallout

Thompson, B., Molina, Y., Viswanath, K., Warnecke, R., & Prelip, M. L. (2016). Strategies to empower communities to reduce health disparities. *Health Affairs (Project Hope)*, *35*(8), 1,424–1,428. https://doi.org/10.1377/hlthaff.2015.1364

Tsai, H. H., Tsai, Y. F., Wang, H. H., Chang, Y. C., & Chu, H. H. (2010). Videoconference program enhances social support, loneliness, and depressive status of elderly nursing home residents. *Aging and Mental Health*, *14*(8), 947–954. https://doi.org/10.1080/13607863.2010.501057

Tsang, H. W., Scudds, R. J., & Chan, E. Y. (2004). Psychosocial impact of SARS. *Emerging Infectious Diseases*, *10*(7), 1,326–1,327. doi:10.3201/eid1007.040090

Xie, X., Xue, Q., Zhou, Y., Zhu, K., Liu, Q., Zhang, J., & Song, R. (2020). Mental health status among children in home confinement during the coronavirus disease 2019 outbreak in Hubei Province, China. *JAMA Pediatrics*. https://doi.org/10.1001/jamapediatrics.2020.1619

Zheng, G., Jimba, M., & Wakai, S. (2005). Exploratory study on psychosocial impact of the severe acute respiratory syndrome (SARS) outbreak on Chinese students living in Japan. *Asia Pacific Journal of Public Health*, *17*(2), 124–129. https://doi.org/10.1177/101053950501700211

# Chapter 6

# How to Support People with Mental Health Conditions During a Pandemic

Jonathan Han Loong Kuek

## Introduction

In 2020, the world waged war against a novel coronavirus (SARS-CoV-2), first discovered at the end of 2019 in Wuhan, China, and responsible for causing the more popularly discussed COVID-19 disease (World Health Organisation [WHO], 2020a). Globally, COVID-19 has killed hundreds of thousands of people, infected millions more, blindsided numerous countries, and demonstrated how the lack of adequate preparations for managing pandemics can lead to devastating societal, economic, and health-related consequences. As countries struggled to contain the rapid transmission of the virus, many chose to implement strict movement restriction and regulatory policies, leaving only essential services operational in order to stem the rate of transmission. These large-scale and radical decisions, whilst necessary, led to major disruptions in the lives of billions globally. Particularly, the lockdowns have severely impacted already vulnerable populations such as individuals with mental health conditions who found themselves in unfamiliar territory and struggled to adapt to the rapidly evolving situation (Chatterjee *et al.*, 2020; Mahase, 2020; Pfefferbaum & North, 2020; Rajkumar, 2020).

There currently exists little robust evidence on the impact of national-level lockdown situations on people with mental health conditions due to the complexities of carrying out research studies during widespread movement restrictions. However, the plethora of case studies, predictive articles, recommendations based on existing literature, as well as short reports emerging during this period have generated a relatively large body of knowledge to draw on. Some examples of potential impacts include the worsening of existing symptoms, heightened levels of stress, anxiety and depressive states, low moods, reluctance to seek help due to fears of contracting the virus, increased suicide risk or ideation, and emergence of new symptoms such as delusions or phobias in relation to the pandemic (Hao *et al.*, 2020; Yao *et al.*, 2020). This chapter discusses important considerations that need to be made when responding to such a crisis, and provides recommendations on how to prepare for such scenarios in the future, in order to mitigate the potential impact of such crisis situations on people experiencing mental health conditions. The main population of focus will be on people with mental health conditions who are living in the community and not in any hospital or residential-type psychiatric settings.

## Inclusion if Community Mental Healthcare in National Response Plans

During a global pandemic, the government oversees and coordinates a nation's response to the situation. This is essential as crises require central and adaptive leadership in order to cope with the rapidly evolving environment, often involving multi-ministerial, multi-sectoral, and multi-agency initiatives (WHO, 2020b). In larger countries, this could also involve multi-state partnerships. As witnessed during COVID-19, mental health responses and preparations were not considered during the initial stages of planning. The WHO's initial guidelines did not consider mental health a top priority during its initial preparedness advisory on 3 February (WHO, 2020b), and it was only brought to attention on 18 March when they released a statement highlighting various mental health and psychosocial considerations (WHO, 2020c). While the focus should undoubtedly be on the necessary steps to reduce the rate and risk of disease transmission, the psychological impact of proposed measures and means of mitigating these consequences should also be considered in tandem.

To do so, a dedicated team of experts from the mental health sector should be included as part of a sub-committee within the national response taskforce whose sole purpose is on managing mental health and psychosocial concerns during the crisis period. This team of experts should constitute members from government, non-governmental services (social service), professional psychiatric or psychological bodies, and private sector organisations, in senior management positions, and ideally with prior experience in managing national-level crisis situations. Doing so would ensure the inclusion of mental health-relevant perspectives and recommendations on how best to implement the various response measures. For example, the state of Massachusetts in the United States (US) recognised the need for a timely mental health response during the early days of COVID-19, and actively engaged the community mental health partners to identify and develop necessary measures (Bartels *et al.*, 2020). This led to emergency policy changes that allocated critical funds, adapted regulations, and refined guidelines necessary to address the challenges of COVID-19. An example of this is the targeted services (e.g., screening of symptoms at local shelters, expedited COVID-19 testing) created for people who were homeless and had a mental health condition.

Conversely, in Singapore, certain mental health and psychological activities such as therapy services were considered non-essential during the introduction of the "circuit-breaker" measure—they were not allowed to operate on their respective premises and therapeutic services had to be conducted virtually (Ministry of Health Singapore [MOH], 2020a; 2020b). This restriction was later revised due to input from the Singapore Psychological Society (SPS) and other mental health advocates, allowing clinicians/therapists working with "unstable and would not benefit from virtual therapy" clients to resume their services (Ong & Meah, 2020). However, this incident demonstrated a clear need for the authorities to place greater emphasis on the unique needs and considerations of people experiencing mental health conditions.

Moving beyond the reactive public health systems, prior pandemics have taught the world important lessons on being proactive and having protocols/frameworks in place which can be activated if necessary. Many countries have adopted some guidelines to inform the decisions made during a crisis. In Singapore, the Disease Outbreak Response System Condition (DORSCON) is an example of such a framework (MOH, 2014). Such preparations should also account for specific mental health guidelines so that a plan of action can be enacted during a pandemic. Looking forward, a toolkit should be conceptualised to contain pertinent information such as the identification of vulnerable populations, best practices, enhanced funding structures, guidelines on services during the crisis, potential psychological impact of the pandemic, to guide a mental health subcommittee in their decision-making processes. By being proactive and anticipatory, the expert team can focus on managing challenges that may not have been predicted. Mental healthcare should not be considered as an afterthought. National response taskforces need to acknowledge and view them as equally important as physiological healthcare. The following segments are potential suggestions that could be included in the toolkit.

## Establishment of Pandemic-Oriented Mental Healthcare Services

Pandemics require new mental health services or initiatives to be launched in order to cope with the atypical environment caused by the measures put in place (i.e., strict movement regulations). A popular option is the establishment of virtual or telephone-based means to provide support for people with mental health conditions during the pandemic period, and many countries have implemented such programmes (Webelhorst *et al.*, 2020; Zhou *et al.*, 2020). For example, in Singapore, the National Care Hotline was launched in April to support the psychological needs of people in the community (Tai, 2020). This hotline was manned by specialist volunteers with training in counselling, crisis management, and other mental health-related disciplines. What is noteworthy is that community mental health organisations were already carrying out such services but did not have the capacity to manage the increased influx of callers who needed support. Hence, the formation of a dedicated mental health pandemic care unit consisting of mental health professionals and volunteers ahead of time is essential.

This newly formed team would only be activated in times of pandemic but should meet regularly and be structured in a similar manner to an organisation. The required key personnel may include management, administrative support, education specialists, logistical support, clinical staff, and a substantial volunteer pool. The team should also aim to include individuals from the government, non-government, and private sectors. Forming such a coalition proactively would allow for potential resources and funding required to sustain operations during a pandemic to be budgeted for, thereby enhancing the quality of support provided.

Upon first notice of a potential pandemic, the team should convene and begin their planning in further consultation with the national mental health advisory subcommittee. A needs assessment (see Kaufman *et al.* (2020) to learn about some of the unique challenges that were identified in relation to COVID-19) of how the mental health community should respond can then be planned out and enacted without delay.

Training and education will play a critical role in the success of this team as the majority of frontline volunteers would be untrained individuals who express interest in supporting the mental health needs of others during a pandemic. A useful tool that can be utilised is the Reflective listening, Assessment of needs, Prioritisation, Intervention, and Disposition (RAPID) model of psychological first aid developed by Johns Hopkins University and designed to support individuals during disaster-type situations (Everly *et al.*, 2012). The strengths of this skillset are that it was designed to be taught to people with no prior training in mental healthcare, can be easily conducted virtually or through a telephone, and provides a rapid but robust first line of defence. Using an established model of care also provides people utilising the service greater confidence in its quality (McDaniel *et al.*, 2014; Rousseau & Gunia, 2017). It is essential that these volunteers are carefully supervised by trained mental health professionals to ensure their well-being and adherence to established protocols based on ethical principles while providing support to others (Howlett & Collins, 2014; Rakovshik *et al.*, 2016; Tackett *et al.*, 2016).

Having such a structure in place allows for cases, which require escalation, to be immediately attended to by a trained mental health professional. Given that funding required for operations would have been planned for, complimentary psychological and mental health services can thus be provided to anyone who needs them during the pandemic period. A similar initiative was started by the Singapore Psychological Society (One Psych Community), where psychologists from the private sector volunteered to reduce their rates or provided free services during the COVID-19 period (Singapore Psychological Society, 2020). With the enactment of a designated mental health pandemic care team, private practice professionals can be employed/compensated under newly established schemes, and provide services during the pandemic period without worrying about the reduction in income from providing pro bono consultations. Taken together, this team could form the basis of a country's main mental health response, supplementing the existing services which may become overwhelmed due to the sudden surge of support requests.

## Broadening and Modification of Existing Mental Healthcare Services

Inevitably, the regular services provided by various mental healthcare organisations will be severely impacted during pandemics. This is further exacerbated by the potential decline their clients may experience due to the new environment they face. Organisations will need to adapt rapidly to deal with these challenges, but also be keenly cognisant of the unique needs of their clients (Ho *et al.*, 2020; Kaufman *et al.*, 2020). As far as possible, changes to their operations should be kept to a minimum whilst ensuring compliance with national regulations relating to service provision. One particularly popular solution was the uptake of virtual or telephone-based consultations during the COVID-19 period (Li *et al.*, 2020; Percudani *et al.*, 2020). However, care must be taken when deciding whether to adopt remote services, and clients should be given the option of face-to-face consultations should they desire. Furthermore, provisions should be made for the option of more frequent follow-ups to be provided to carefully monitor the client's condition during and after the pandemic period. Alternatively, referrals should be made to complementary services such as care hotlines or other community-based services if the organisation is unable to manage an increased workload.

Furthermore, due to movement restrictions often enacted during pandemics, community teams need to be strengthened and expanded to ensure their ability to manage the caseload is preserved. Coupled with the shift towards remote service provision, these teams may need to conduct home-based visits more frequently due to their clients' worsening condition or in the case of a crisis where an individual is suicidal. This involves greater collaboration with similar agencies, restructuring of roles, and a redirection of necessary resources such as funding and logistical requirements to support these efforts. Identification of vulnerable populations within the mental health spectrum, such as individuals with an addiction condition or those who face family issues on a regular basis (Holmes *et al.*, 2020), could also aid in allocating assistance to people who may need it more urgently.

Mental health organisations and departments will also need to direct a certain amount of resources to support frontline medical and administrative staff such as nurses, temperature screeners, and doctors who are dealing directly with the pandemic. It is well documented that these healthcare professionals are at a greater risk of facing burnout, elevated stress levels, and poorer mental health states during such crises (Greenberg *et al.*, 2020; Tan *et al.*, 2020). Hence, these mental health units/teams require prior training in grief and crisis management to ensure that they can tackle the unique issues these frontline healthcare workers face. Such a setup should be prepared by hospitals beforehand, and be activated during pandemics. Doing so allows for ample time to carefully select and train mental health professionals who are suitable candidates in taking on such a role.

It is also pertinent that mental health professionals are cared for during pandemics. Given the sudden increase in workload, constantly facing death, and the various adaptations they are required to make, it can cause uncertainty and anxiety in these professionals as well (Galbraith *et al.*, 2020; Maben & Bridges, 2020). One useful solution could be the utilisation of peer support programmes (Jadwisiak, 2020). The concept of peer support rests on the notion that people going through similarly challenging situations are best positioned to help others who need assistance. However, before peer support programmes are implemented, an understanding on the willingness to utilise such initiatives must be established. Every organisation has a different culture and operating procedure, making it crucial that these factors are carefully studied and understood before any modification to the status quo is made.

## Recovery Oriented Approach

Underpinning the various proposed changes should be an adherence to recovery-oriented principles of mental healthcare. The recovery-oriented approach promotes acceptance of experiences associated with mental illness as part of a person's developmental journey and the idea that living a fulfilling life is possible with or without continued symptoms of mental illness (Davidson *et al.*, 2006; Slade, 2010; Symanski-Tondora *et al.*, 2014; Xie, 2013). Such an approach encourages clinicians and practitioners to take a step back and allow their clients to share what they believe is necessary to support their recovery. Conversely, traditional clinical notions towards mental healthcare view them as illnesses, as clusters of symptoms that need to be eradicated for people to resume their regular functions (Jacob, 2015).

Recovery-oriented approaches also emphasise the need for empowerment (Hunt & Resnick, 2015; Schwartz *et al.*, 2013), goal setting (Clarke *et al.*, 2012), and regaining a sense of self-determination (Andresen *et al.*, 2006). This can be achieved through shared decision-making processes where the client and clinician make choices together about the types of treatment or care management that the client receives. Having the choice and the ability to decide for themselves are key aspects of the recovery-oriented approach (Smith & Williams, 2016; Zisman-Ilani *et al.*, 2017). This can be translated to practice by providing an ample selection of options, and clinicians need to make the extra and conscious effort to educate and inform their clients about the pros and cons of each choice, so that they are able to make an informed and appropriate decision.

Furthermore, recovery-oriented interventions such as the Wellness Recovery Action Plan (or WRAP; see Copeland (2002) for how to create and use one) can be especially useful during pandemic situations as they are self-directed and require minimal input from mental health professionals. However, a new plan should be created at the start of the pandemic with potential movement restrictions in mind, as the activities and response options will need to cater for the environment that people find themselves in. Existing WRAPs will also need to be revisited to ensure that they are still relevant and able to continue providing support to the well-being of people with mental health conditions during pandemics.

A noteworthy point is that adopting recovery-oriented approaches can be challenging in the beginning due to the reversal of power dynamics between a clinician and their client. However, allowing people to decide how they want to be supported is the foundation for a trusting and nurturing partnership. This is particularly important during pandemic situations as every individuals' needs will be different, due in part to their reactions to the new environments they find themselves in. Only by carefully listening and understanding these unique needs can clinicians provide the adequate types and levels of support to people experiencing mental health conditions.

# Conclusion

Pandemics constitute great threats to societies experiencing them, and vulnerable populations such as people with mental health conditions are particularly susceptible to the negative impact accompanying these crises. This chapter has provided a simple illustration of how mental health perspectives can be woven into larger pandemic responses. By being proactive and creative, national strategies can potentially mitigate some of the unseen consequences derived from the various restrictions often put in place to contain the transmission of a virus. It is crucial that mental health experts are involved during the planning of a national response so that the necessary steps to reduce the negative impact of these regulations can be introduced. It is important to note that each country will need to adapt the recommendations to their cultural context and societal needs. More importantly, mental healthcare should not be an afterthought during a country's response to pandemics and must be considered alongside any potential plans to tackle them.

# Acknowledgement

The views expressed in this chapter are the author's only and do not represent the official position or view of the University of Sydney, or any organisation he is affiliated with.

# Editors' Note

In July 2020, a dedicated website with various resources on mental health, mindline.sg, was launched to help users assess their well-being and match them with forms of assistance if needed (Yip, 2020). The introduction of such initiatives (e.g., mindline.sg, National Care Hotline) would definitely help Singaporeans get the mental health assistance that they need easily and conveniently.

# References

Andresen, R., Caputi, P., & Oades, L. (2006). Stages of recovery instrument: Development of a measure of recovery from serious mental illness. *Australian and New Zealand Journal of Psychiatry, 40*(11–12), 972–980. https://doi.org/10.1080/j.1440-1614.2006.01921.x

Bartels, S. J., Baggett, T. P., Freudenreich, O., & Bird, B. L. (2020) Case study of Massachusetts COVID-19 emergency policy reforms to support community-based behavioral health and reduce mortality of people with serious mental illness. *Psychiatric Services*. Advance online publication. https://doi.org/10.1176/appi.ps.202000244

Chatterjee, S., Barikar C. M., & Mukherjee, A. (2020). Impact of COVID-19 pandemic on pre-existing mental health problems. *Asian Journal of Psychiatry, 51*, 102071. https://doi.org/10.1016/j.ajp.2020.102071

Clarke, S., Oades, L. G., & Crowe, T. P. (2012). Recovery in mental health: A movement towards well-being and meaning in contrast to an avoidance of symptoms. *Psychiatric Rehabilitation Journal, 35*(4), 297–304. https://doi.org/10.2975/35.4.2012.297.304

Copeland, M. E. (2002). Wellness recovery action plan: A system for monitoring, reducing and eliminating uncomfortable or dangerous physical symptoms and emotional feelings. *Occupational Therapy in Mental Health, 17*(3–4), 127–150. https://doi.org/10.1300/J004v17n03_09

Davidson, L., O'Connell, M., Tondora, J., Styron, T., & Kangas, K. (2006). The top ten concerns about recovery encountered in mental health system transformation. *Psychiatric Services, 57*(5), 640–645. https://doi.org/10.1176/appi.ps.57.5.640

Everly, G. S., Barnett, D. J., & Links, J. M. (2012). The Johns Hopkins model of psychological first aid (RAPID-PFA): Curriculum development and content validation. *International Journal of Emergency Mental Health, 14*(2), 95–103.

Galbraith, N., Boyda, D., Mcfeeters, D., & Hassan, T. (2020). The mental health of doctors during the Covid-19 pandemic. *BJPsych Bulletin.* Advance online publication. 1–7. https://doi.org/10.1192/bjb.2020.44

Greenberg, N., Docherty, M., Gnanapragasam, S., & Wessely, S. (2020). Managing mental health challenges faced by healthcare workers during Covid-19 pandemic. *BMJ, 368*, m1211. https://doi.org/10.1136/bmj.m1211

Hao, F., Tan, W., Jiang, L., Zhang, L., Zhao, X., Zou, Y., Hu, Y., Luo, X., Jiang, X., McIntyre, R. S., Tran, B., Sun, J., Zhang, Z., Ho, R., Ho C., & Tam, W. (2020). Do psychiatric patients experience more psychiatric symptoms during COVID-19 pandemic and lockdown? A case-control study with service and research implications for immunopsychiatry. *Brain, Behavior, and Immunity.* https://doi.org/10.1016/j.bbi.2020.04.069

Ho, C., Chee, C., & Ho, R. (2020). Mental health strategies to combat the psychological impact of COVID-19 beyond paranoia and panic. *Annals of the Academy of Medicine, Singapore, 49*(3), 155–160. http://search.proquest.com/docview/2381848739/

Holmes, E. A., O'Connor, R. C., Perry, V. H., Tracey, I., Wessely, S., Arseneault, L., Ballard, C., Christensen, H., Silver, R. C., Everall, I., Ford, T., John, A.,

Kabir, T., King, K., Madan, I., Michie, S., Przybylski, A. L., Shafran, R., ... Bullmore, E. (2020). Multidisciplinary research priorities for the COVID-19 pandemic: A call for action for mental health science. *The Lancet Psychiatry*, *7*(6), 547–560. https://doi.org/10.1016/S2215-0366(20)30168-1

Howlett, S., & Collins, A. (2014). Vicarious traumatisation: Risk and resilience among crisis support volunteers in a community organisation. *South African Journal of Psychology*, *44*(2), 180–190. https://doi.org/10.1177/008124-6314524387

Hunt, M. G., & Resnick, S. G. (2015). Two birds, one stone: Unintended consequences and a potential solution for problems with recovery in mental health. *Psychiatric Services*, *66*(11), 1,235–1,237. https://doi:10.1176/appi.ps.201400518

Jacob, K. S. (2015). Recovery model of mental illness: A complementary approach to psychiatric care. *Indian Journal of Psychological Medicine*, *37*(2), 117–119. https://doi:10.4103/0253-7176.155605

Jadwisiak, M. (2020). Peer support — A secret weapon in the fight against COVID-19. *Mental Health Weekly*, *30*(19), 5. https://doi.org/10.1002/mhw.32357

Kaufman, K. R., Petkova, E., Bhui, K. S., & Schulze, T. G. (2020). A global needs assessment in times of a global crisis: world psychiatry response to the COVID-19 pandemic. *BJPsych Open*, *6*(3), e48. https://doi.org/10.1192/bjo.2020.25

Li, W., Yang, Y., Liu, Z., Zhao, Y., Zhang, Q., Zhang, L., Cheung, T., & Xiang Y. (2020). Progression of mental health services during the COVID-19 outbreak in China. *International Journal of Biological Sciences*, *16*(10), 1,732–1,738. https://doi.org/10.7150/ijbs.45120

Maben, J., & Bridges, J. (2020). Covid-19: Supporting nurses' psychological and mental health. *Journal of Clinical Nursing*. Advance online publication. https://doi.org/10.1111/jocn.15307

Mahase, E. (2020). Covid-19: Mental health consequences of pandemic need urgent research, paper advises. *BMJ*, *369*, m1515. https://doi.org/10.1136/bmj.m1515

McDaniel, S. H., Grus, C. L., Cubic, B. A., Hunter, C. L., Kearney, L. K., Schuman, C. C., Karel, M. J., Kessler, R. S., Larkin, K. T., McCutcheon, S., Miller, B. F., Nash, J., Qualls, S. H., Connolly, K. S., Stancin, T., Stanton, A. L., Sturm, L. A., & Johnson, S. B. (2014). Competencies for psychology practice in primary care. *American Psychologist*, *69*(4), 409–429. https://doi.org/10.1037/a0036072

Ministry of Health. (2014). *Being prepared for a pandemic.* https://perma.cc/28SV-XRUA

Ministry of Health. (2020a). *Continuation of essential healthcare services during period of heightened safe distancing measures.* https://perma.cc/UCR5-5SXA

Ministry of Health. (2020b). *Continuation of essential healthcare services during period of heightened safe distancing measures (Annex A)*. https://perma.cc/U9TV-HDLW

Ong, J., & Meah, N. (2020, April 07). Covid-19: Impact on mental health under the spotlight, as MOH clarifies stance on treatment amid "circuit breaker". *Today Online*. https://perma.cc/R5XD-DQ7H

Percudani, M., Corradin, M., Moreno, M., Indelicato, A., & Vita, A. (2020). Mental health services in Lombardy during COVID-19 outbreak. *Psychiatry Research, 288*, 112980. https://doi.org/10.1016/j.psychres.2020.112980

Pfefferbaum, B., & North, C. (2020). Mental health and the Covid-19 pandemic. *The New England Journal of Medicine*. https://doi.org/10.1056/NEJMp2008017

Rajkumar, R. P. (2020). COVID-19 and mental health: A review of existing literature. *Asian Journal of Psychiatry, 52,* 102066. https://doi.org/10.1016/j.ajp.2020.102066

Rakovshik, S., McManus, F., Vazquez-Montes, M., Muse, K., & Ougrin, D. (2016). Is supervision necessary? Examining the effects of internet-based CBT training with and without supervision. *Journal of Consulting and Clinical Psychology, 84*(3), 191–199. https://doi.org/10.1037/ccp0000079

Rousseau, D., & Gunia, B. (2017). Evidence-based practice: The psychology of EBP implementation. *Annual Review of Psychology, 67*(1), 667–692. https://doi.org/10.1146/annurev-psych-122414-033336

Schwartz, R., Estein, O., Komaroff, J., Lamb, J., Myers, M., Stewart, J., Park, M. (2013). Mental health consumers and providers dialogue in an institutional setting: A participatory approach to promoting recovery-oriented care. *Psychiatric Rehabilitation Journal, 36*(2), 113–115. https://doi.org/10.1037/h0094980

Singapore Psychological Society. (2020). *One psych community tackling the Covid-19 crisis*. https://perma.cc/YTD8-BDKL

Slade, M. (2010). Mental illness and well-being: The central importance of positive psychology and recovery approaches. *BMC Health Services Research, 10*(1), 26. https://doi.org/10.1186/1472-6963-10-26

Smith, G. P., & Williams, T. M. (2016). From providing a service to being of service: Advances in person-centred care in mental health. *Current Opinion in Psychiatry, 29*(5), 292–297. https://doi.org/10.1097/YCO.0000000000000264

Symanski-Tondora, J. L., Miller, R., Slade, M., & Davidson, L. (2014). *Partnering for recovery in mental health: A practical guide to person-centered planning* (2nd ed.). Chichester, West Sussex, UK: Hoboken, NJ.

Tackett, M. J., Nash, L., Stucky, K. J., & Nierenberg, B. (2016). Supervision in rehabilitation psychology: Application of Beatrice Wright's value-laden beliefs and principles. *Rehabilitation Psychology, 61*(1), 74–81. https://doi.org/10.1037/rep0000070

Tai, J. (2020, April 11). Coronavirus: National Care Hotline now open, manned by 300 volunteers. *The Straits Times.* https://perma.cc/MN9R-5LXD

Tan, B. Y. Q., Chew, N. W, S,, Lee, G. K. H., Jing, M., Goh, Y., Yeo, L. L. L., Zhang, K., Khan, F. A., Shanmugam, G. N., Chan, B. P. L., Sunny, S., Chandra, B., Ong, J. J. Y., Paliwal, P. R., Wong, L. Y. H., Sagayanathan, R., Chen, J. T., Ng, A. Y. Y., Teoh, H. L., … Sharma, V. K. (2020). Psychological Impact of the COVID-19 Pandemic on Health Care Workers in Singapore. *Annals of Internal Medicine.* Advance online publication. https://doi.org/10.7326/M20-1083

Webelhorst, C., Jepsen, L., & Rummel-Kluge, C. (2020). Utilization of e-mental-health and online self-management interventions of patients with mental disorders-A cross-sectional analysis. *PLoS ONE, 15*(4), e0231373. https://doi.org/10.1371/journal.pone.0231373

World Health Organisation. (2020a). *Naming the coronavirus disease (COVID-19) and the virus that causes it.* https://www.who.int/emergencies/diseases/novel-coronavirus-2019/technical-guidance/naming-the-coronavirus-disease-(covid-2019)-and-the-virus-that-causes-it

World Health Organisation. (2020b). *2019 Novel coronavirus (2019-nCoV): Strategic preparedness and response plan.* https://www.who.int/docs/default-source/coronaviruse/srp-04022020.pdf

World Health Organisation. (2020c). *Mental health and psychosocial considerations during the COVID-19 outbreak.* https://www.who.int/publications-detail/WHO-2019-nCoV-MentalHealth-2020.1

Xie, H. (2013). Strengths-based approach for mental health recovery. *Iranian Journal of Psychiatry and Behavioral Sciences, 7*(2), 5–10.

Yao, H., Chen, J., & Xu, Y. (2020). Patients with mental health disorders in the COVID-19 epidemic. *The Lancet Psychiatry, 7*(4), e21. https://doi.org/10.1016/S2215-0366(20)30090-0

Yip, C. (2020, July 7). COVID-19: One-stop mental health platform launched to match users with resources and helplines. *Channel News Asia.* https://www.channelnewsasia.com/news/singapore/covid-19-mental-health-platform-launched-mindline-sg-12909640

Zhou, X., Snoswell, C. L., Harding, L. E., Bambling, M., Edirippulige, S., Bai, X., & Smith, A. C. (2020). The role of telehealth in reducing the mental health burden from COVID-19. *Telemedicine and e-Health, 26*(4), 377–379. https://doi.org/10.1089/tmj.2020.0068

Zisman-Ilani, Y., Barnett, E., Harik, J., Pavlo, A., & O'Connell, M. (2017). Expanding the concept of shared decision making for mental health: Systematic search and scoping review of interventions. *The Mental Health Review, 22*(3), 191–213. https://doi.org/10.1108/MHRJ-01-2017-0002

# Chapter 7

# Coping with COVID-19: The Role of Religion in Times of Crisis

Jonathan E. Ramsay

## Introduction

The most serious pandemic of the globalised age has had tremendous consequences, both physical and psychological, for the world's population. Few people have remained unaffected, although it is undeniable that certain individuals and groups have suffered more than others. Many journalists and medical professionals have highlighted the disproportionately high mortality rates among ethnic minorities in several nations (Pareek *et al.*, 2020), while others have decried the severity of the psychological impact that social distancing has had on individuals struggling with mental health issues (Yao *et al.*, 2020). There can be no doubt that COVID-19 is everyone's problem. Yet, it is vitally important to mitigate and leverage differences in vulnerability and resilience respectively if we are to minimise the total cost of this terrible illness.

The psychology of religion can offer important insights into why some individuals and groups struggle more than others in coping with the impacts of COVID-19. Why do some people cope better with loss and bereavement than others? Why do some individuals flout social distancing laws when the majority comply? And why do times of crisis bring out the best in some people while others retreat into bigotry and division? These are just some of the questions that research in the psychology of religion—as well as other areas of psychology and the wider human and behavioural sciences—can help to answer.

In no place is this better exemplified than in the area of religious coping: "a specific mode of coping that is inherently derived from religious beliefs, practices, experiences, emotions, or relationships" (Abu-Raiya & Pargament, 2015, p. 25). Building on Lazarus and Folkman (1984)'s general coping theory, research in religious coping seeks to examine how religious and spiritual resources can be mobilised as a coping response to stresses in the environment, such as the loss or threat of loss during a pandemic. This chapter seeks to apply important findings in the religious and spiritual coping literature to the local, regional, and global fight against COVID-19 and potentially similar future outbreaks.

While much of the extant research in the field has been conducted in Christian populations in North America and Europe, a significant number of scholars are now redressing this imbalance by examining such questions in other religious groups and cultural contexts (Abu-Raiya & Pargament, 2015). Asia, and particularly Southeast Asia, have been at the forefront of these developments, owning in no small part to the incredible richness and diversity of religious beliefs in this part of the world (Brennan, 2014). While subtle differences are inevitable, it also seems that religious belief and affiliation do have some consistent implications for thought, feeling, and behaviour. This is reassuring for researchers and policymakers seeking to leverage the global academic output when planning and implementing evidence-based interventions based on religious coping.

The list of findings and recommendations covered in this chapter is not exhaustive. Nevertheless, it does focus on the most well-established findings, as well as those that translate most readily into actionable policy changes. While some may be more appropriate in certain jurisdictions, it is hoped that researchers, practitioners, and policymakers can all derive some valuable insights from the key points contained herein.

## Religion, the Search for Meaning, and Well-Being

Religious beliefs provide answers to existential questions; they are a framework for deriving meaning from life experiences in the absence of proof that such meaning truly exists. This property and function of religious belief has long been acknowledged by philosophers and theologians alike (Neville, 2018), and pervades the language used by religious believers to describe their lives and their attempts to make sense of them (Fletcher, 2004). When confronting the big issues—such as morality, life and death, purpose, and creation—religious individuals can take comfort from a set of beliefs, shared among fellow adherents, that provide a sense of certainty and significance. While different religions diverge significantly in their teachings on existential issues such as free will, the afterlife, and the means by which salvation can be achieved, they are united in their view that our lives, and the way they are lived, actually matter. This has profound implications for the way that religious believers interpret and respond to events throughout their lives.

One of the most well-established findings in the psychology of religion is the positive association between religiousness and well-being (Koenig *et al.*, 2012). Religious individuals tend to be happier and more fulfilled than those who do not identify as religious, although spirituality outside of organised religions has also been found to engender similar benefits (Ivtzan *et al.*, 2013). The ability to derive meaning has been identified as a possible link in the causal chain between religion and enhanced well-being (Steger & Frazier, 2005), along with other potential mediators such as positive emotions and need satisfaction that will be discussed in subsequent sections. While research has shown that religious individuals see divine purpose and significance in day-to-day events (Ramsay *et al.*, 2018), this ability to derive meaning is even more striking in the case of highly impactful events (Lupfer *et al.*, 1996). This suggests that religion should serve a psychologically protective function when confronted with an unprecedented global emergency such as COVID-19.

Research has shown that religious individuals often invoke divine forces and will when seeking to explain negative, unanticipated, and highly impactful events such as natural disasters (Riggio *et al.*, 2018). While this has previously been investigated in the context of earthquakes (Sibley & Bulbulia, 2012), and hurricanes (Aten *et al.*, 2012), pandemics such as COVID-19 seem likely to function in a similar way. Associating such terrible events with divine will or purpose may seem like a recipe for spiritual crisis, yet ostensibly negative explanations (from a psychological sense) may nevertheless serve an important purpose. Some scholars have gone so far as to suggest that the prevalence of natural disasters may play an important role in maintaining or enhancing aggregate religiosity over time (Bentzen, 2019), as less religious individuals turn to religion to help them explain events that otherwise seem inexplicable. This is the essence of religious coping, one of the most widely researched topics in the psychology of religion.

## Religious Coping

This use of religion—as a coping mechanism to deal with hardship and adversity—is widespread among members of many different faiths. Unsurprisingly, religious coping is positively associated with religiosity, with those who are more religious utilising religious coping methods more than those who are less religious (Harrison *et al.*, 2001). Differences also exist between religious groups (Bhui *et al.*, 2008), with members of the Abrahamic, monotheistic faiths (e.g., Christianity, Islam, Judaism) employing it more than adherents of Eastern religions (e.g., Buddhism, Hinduism, Taoism). Religious coping is also heterogeneous, in that certain religious coping methods or strategies are psychologically beneficial and lead to better outcomes, whereas others have a detrimental effect. This key distinction between positive and negative religious coping is a fundamental one, and has been documented across many different cultural and religious groups (Abu-Raiya & Pargament, 2015).

Positive religious coping encompasses strategies that allow an individual to maintain (1) a secure and positive relationship with their God(s) or the divine, (2) belief that there is greater meaning to be found, and (3) a sense of spiritual kinship and connection with other people (Abu-Raiya & Pargament, 2015). Such strategies include benevolent reappraisals, in which the negative event is reappraised as serving a positive purpose (e.g., strengthening faith, spiritual growth), and seeking spiritual support, in which the negative event prompts the individual to seek comfort in their relationship with the divine. These coping methods and others like them have been found to serve a protective function, buffering believers against the worst psychological consequences of the negative experience (Pargament *et al.*, 1998). Employment of positive religious coping strategies has been found to predict better psychological adjustment across many different studies, although the majority of these have been conducted in Western Christian populations (Ano & Vasconcelles, 2005).

Negative religious coping represents the opposing possibility, that religious coping strategies may weaken relationships with the divine, call meaning into question, and disrupt relationships with other people. Such strategies often represent the negative mirror image of a corresponding positive religious coping strategy (e.g., punishing reappraisals, interpersonal religious discontent), but can also represent a distinctive approach (e.g., demonic reappraisal; in which the event is attributed to evil spirits or other malevolent supernatural forces). Negative religious coping strategies have unsurprisingly been found to exhibit a negative relationship with mental health outcomes (Faigin *et al.*, 2014; Lee *et al.*, 2013), although evidence gathered across a variety of different contexts and populations indicate that negative religious coping is significantly less prevalent than positive religious coping (Harrison *et al.*, 2001). This would explain the net positive association between religion and well-being, despite evidence that the relationship may be negative for some individuals under certain circumstances (Lau & Ramsay, 2019).

## *Islamic Religious Coping*

As in many other areas of the psychology of religion, the elephant in the room of religious coping is the cross-cultural replicability of the key findings and the cross-cultural validity of the key measures. The lion's share of religious coping research has been conducted in Christian populations in North America (Abu-Raiya & Pargament, 2015), although the past decade has seen a significant increase in the volume of published research examining religious coping among Muslims, often conducted by scholars based in Asia (e.g., Khan *et al.*, 2012; Nurasikin *et al.*, 2013). These studies are an important extension beyond those that examine religious coping among minority or immigrant groups in Western contexts. While such research is still relatively rare, it has already uncovered some interesting differences and nuances in the way religious coping manifests across different religious groups and affiliations.

One consistent finding is that Muslims tend to report using positive religious coping methods more than Christian populations (Abu-Raiya & Pargament, 2015), although there remains the possibility that this may reflect religious differences in the acceptability of expressing doubts regarding faith or disagreement with religious authorities (Banu, 2020). Further work will be required to tease apart these different possibilities. A recent study of Muslim youth in Indonesia found that positive religious coping protects against loneliness (French *et al.*, 2020), while a multinational study of Islamic religious coping, which included a Malaysian sample, found that positive religious coping predicted better satisfaction with life but did not predict lower depression (Abu-Raiya *et al.*, 2019). Interestingly, reported levels of positive religious coping and the strength of its association with satisfaction with life were greatest among the Malaysian sample. Specific investigations of Islamic religious coping outside of Southeast Asia's three Muslim-majority nations are rare, although qualitative (Hassan & Mehta, 2010) and quantitative studies (Banu, 2020) suggest the importance of religious coping strategies among Muslims in countries where Islam is a minority religion.

One hallmark of the nascent Islamic religious coping literature is the occasional presence of unexpected relationships between positive religious coping and various outcomes. While Khan *et al.* (2016) observed unexpectedly positive relationship between positive religious coping and distress in a sample of Pakistani Muslims, the same authors (Khan *et al.*, 2011) also found a positive relationship between positive religious coping and poorer psychological functioning in a sample of Pakistani Muslim hospital patients. However, given that both these studies used the same method of measuring coping, there remains a possibility that these findings could be specific to the measure used. The need to adapt and validate more detailed measures of non-Christian religious coping, as well as to replicate findings across multiple measures, is a pressing concern in the study of non-Christian religious coping.

It has also been documented across several studies that negative religious coping, although less widely reported among Muslims, is equally, if not more, predictive of relevant mental health outcomes (Banu, 2020; Gardner *et al.*, 2014). Tentative evidence suggests that spiritual discontent—the form of negative religious coping pertaining to confusion over divine purpose and dissatisfaction with the quality of the relationship with the divine agent—may be predictive of worsened mental health outcomes for Muslims (Banu, 2020). Researchers have also found evidence for greater death anxiety, obsession, and depressive symptoms among Muslims that employ negative religious coping (Mohammadzadeh & Najafi, 2018). These findings suggest a need to identify instances of negative religious coping with crises among Muslims, and to intervene in such a way that positive religious coping strategies are encouraged.

## *Religious Coping in Eastern Religions*

The literature surrounding religious coping among Buddhists and Hindus is sparse. The little research that has been conducted often involves minority samples from Western nations, a problem previously noted by Abu-Raiya and Pargament (2015). There has been a notable improvement in the past few years, with studies conducted in Buddhist majority nations such as Sri Lanka (de Zoysa & Wickrama, 2011) and Singapore (Xu, 2019), as well as nations with strong Buddhist cultural influence such as China (Pan *et al.*, 2017) and South Korea (Noh *et al.*, 2016).

In an important early quantitative study, Phillips *et al.* (2012) developed a measure of Buddhist religious coping (the BCOPE), which comprises 14 distinct coping strategies: 10 that can be characterised as positive religious coping, three that represent negative religious coping, and one that is mixed or ambivalent in its implications. The positive religious coping factors were generally found to be related to better psychological adjustment, whereas the negative religious coping factors were associated with worse outcomes. Similar results were observed in a sample of palliative care providers by Falb and Pargament (2013). Unfortunately, this method of measurement has not been widely used and has not yet been validated (i.e., checked for appropriateness and functionality) outside the Western Buddhist context in which it was developed. Such research is an urgent priority if religious coping is to be leveraged in response to major regional crises such as COVID-19.

Studies of Buddhist coping in Asia tend to be either qualitative (e.g., de Zoysa & Wickrama, 2011; Xu, 2019), or use general religious coping measures that do not take into account the major theological differences between Buddhism and monotheistic faiths (e.g., Noh *et al.*, 2016). Evidence from qualitative research suggests some similarity with Christian and Islamic religious coping (e.g., positive coping methods that rely on finding meaning in adversity), yet also highlights stark differences in the reliance on meditative coping and ego transcendence (Xu, 2019). Further research will be required to construct appropriate measures of these coping practices, with a view to documenting their prevalence and effectiveness in dealing with stress and trauma. Researchers should also take inspiration from qualitative research on Buddhist coping in the aftermath of the 2004 Indian Ocean Tsunami (e.g., Falk, 2012; Silva, 2006), with a view to incorporating these insights into new measures of Buddhist coping.

Studies of religious coping in other Eastern religious traditions are even more rare. Tarakeshwar *et al.* (2003) conducted one of the few explicit examinations of Hindu religious coping, developing and initially validating a measure comprising three sub-scales—God-focused coping, spirituality-focused coping, and religious guilt, anger, and passivity—with the first two associated with better mental health outcomes and the third being associated with poorer functioning. As with the BCOPE, this measure has not been widely used since its development and suffers from the limitation of having been developed in a relatively small sample of American Hindus that are unrepresentative of the larger corpus of the Hindu faith.

Studies of religious coping in Asian Hindus have tended to assume the applicability and validity of religious coping measures developed for use in American Christian populations. Pandey and Singh (2019) examined positive religious coping in a sample of Indian community health activists, observing a buffering effect with respect to the detrimental effects of work-family conflict, while Grover *et al.* (2016) found evidence of increased negative religious coping and decreased positive religious coping among self-harm attempters in India. While such studies are important, it is regrettable that only one study to date has attempted to characterise the forms and aspects of religious coping that are unique to Hinduism, or attempted to draw parallels with other Eastern religions such as Buddhism.

## Implications and Recommendations

The literature surveyed in the preceding section is notable for its imbalance. Nevertheless, while most of the research on religious coping has focused on Western Christian samples, there is scope for the application of the resulting findings. The present section will summarise the key findings to date with respect to religious coping in Southeast Asian populations, before making five recommendations for policy and practice considering the risks posed by COVID-19 and possible future pandemics.

One clear convergence in the literature is the distinction between positive and negative religious coping. Across different religions, it seems that some religious coping practices are psychologically beneficial whereas others are harmful. Another consistent thread is the importance of views of the divine—specifically whether God(s) are deemed to be benevolent or punitive—although this is likely to be more important (and certainly more straightforward) in the Abrahamic faiths than in Eastern religions. It is also true that reliance on religious coping varies substantially across religious populations, with groups characterised by greater religiosity employing it to a greater extent that those exhibiting lower religiosity. It is therefore important that interventions seek to enhance positive religious coping and reduce negative religious coping, particularly among groups characterised by high religiosity. The negative impact of future pandemics on collective mental health may be lessened if these general principles are used to guide the development of policy and practice.

Enactment of these general principles will nevertheless require specific actions. Below are five recommendations for leveraging religious coping in the fight against COVID-19 and future pandemics.

## *Recommendation 1: Encourage Development of Religious and Spiritual Competencies*

There is a clear disconnect between the prevalence of religious coping and the secularised nature of mental health service delivery in many countries. If religious belief provides both a framework for interpreting trauma and a toolkit for responding to it, then it is important for mental health practitioners to be (1) comfortable discussing religious and spiritual matters with their clients, and (2) sufficiently knowledgeable of major religions to be able to productively (and sensitively) engage in such discussions.

There have been longstanding calls for greater recognition of religious and spiritual issues in psychotherapy (e.g., Zinnbauer & Pargament, 2000), and recent attempts in Western settings to develop a training programme for developing related competencies (Pearce *et al.*, 2019). Such efforts are aligned with a wider movement towards recognising and respecting diversity in mental health settings, as well as considering the specific needs of minority groups in treatment (Mayer *et al.*, 2008). While this movement has gained the greatest traction in the West, there is an increasing recognition of this need in Southeast Asia (Suthendran, 2017). As such, governments and relevant professional bodies should conduct a religious and spiritual competency needs analysis for the mental health services, with a view to developing a training programme that develops these skills and competencies.

## Recommendation 2: Attend to the Risks Associated with Negative Religious Coping

Although there is much work to be done in replicating and consolidating key findings in the religious coping literature, a consistent theme is that negative religious coping predicted worsened mental health outcomes. The limited research on negative religious coping in the regional context also suggests that the links with mental health seem stronger.

Mental health professionals equipped with the aforementioned religious and spiritual competencies should therefore be particularly watchful for the presence of negative religious coping strategies such as punishing God reappraisals and spiritual discontent, which have been implicated in worsened mental health in both Christians (Pargament *et al.*, 2000) and Muslims (Ghorbani *et al.*, 2016). Such strategies are more likely to manifest in anxious individuals with personalities that predispose them to rumination and worry (Lau & Ramsay, 2019; Silton *et al.*, 2014). It is therefore recommended that policymakers and practitioners, working with religious authorities, strive to develop and pilot test interventions designed to reduce negative religious coping.

## Recommendation 3: Recognise the Social Aspects of Positive Religious Coping

The need to affiliate and belong is thought to be a key component of religious experience (Graham & Haidt, 2010), and it should come as no surprise that many religious coping methods—particularly the positive ones—involve seeking and gaining support from the religious community. This is well-established in both Christian and Islamic religious coping (Abu-Raiya & Pargament, 2015), although while this remains an empirical question for members of Eastern religions, it is hard to imagine this aspect of religious coping being unimportant.

This represents something of a conundrum when dealing with a pandemic. On the one hand, religious communities provide critical coping resources for individuals coping with personal loss or more generalised distress; yet on the other hand, religious congregation has been heavily implicated in the spread of the virus in several Southeast Asian nations (Pung *et al.*, 2020; Quadri, 2020). To balance these concerns, elected officials and policymakers should work with religious authorities to provide and champion alternative methods of social support (e.g., video conferencing, online social networks) when large physical gatherings are prohibited.

## Recommendation 4: Remove Barriers to Discussing Religion in Healthcare Settings

Training mental health professionals to be comfortable and competent in discussing religious and spiritual matters only addresses one part of a complex issue. It has been documented that religious individuals can be reluctant to discuss matters of faith in non-religious settings (Pirutinsky *et al.*, 2009), although other research suggests that many patients desire such discussions yet feel unable to have them (Best *et al.*, 2015; Williams *et al.*, 2011).

These issues can be exacerbated in secular multi-religious societies where clear demarcations between religion and the public sphere have been deemed necessary to avoid religious enmity and conflict (Thio, 2009). While it is necessary to tread lightly when considering the discussion of religion in traditionally secular spaces, collaborations between healthcare providers and religious bodies may reduce the perception that religious discussions should be restricted to the temple, mosque, or church. In turn, this would facilitate referral from religious counselling services to mental health service providers.

## Recommendation 5: Enhance Research in Understudied Populations

While there do seem to be common coping themes that run across religious groups, there are likely to be at least as many divergences. Assessing the extent of consistency or inconsistency will not be possible until more religious coping research is conducted in understudied religious groups, particularly Hindus, Sikhs, Buddhists, and Taoists. This is especially important in Southeast Asia, which exhibits a tremendous religious diversity both across and within nations (Brennan, 2014), as well as a prevalence of non-doctrinal folk religion and incorporation of elements from other faiths (Sinha, 2008). Psychologists interested in facilitating the development of evidence-based interventions based on religious coping will need to adopt a more contextualised approach if they are to cater to the populations of Southeast Asia.

# Conclusion

It is widely recognised that we will be living with the SARS-CoV-2 virus for the foreseeable future (Denworth, 2020), and the risk of pandemics more generally has been brought into sharp focus by the previously unimaginable suffering and disruption caused by COVID-19. Psychology and the behavioural sciences have a critical role to play in mitigating the spread of such diseases and helping people to live with their consequences, yet these contributions will only be possible through partnerships with practitioners, policymakers, and religious leaders. Religious coping can be a powerful tool to promote resilience in individuals and communities, but effective implementation will require a collaborative and joined-up approach to mental health service provision. This may be the silver lining to the dark cloud of COVID-19.

# References

Abu-Raiya, H., & Pargament, K. I. (2015). Religious coping among diverse religions: Commonalities and divergences. *Psychology of Religion and Spirituality*, *7*(1), 24–33. https://doi.org/10.1037/a0037652

Abu-Raiya, H., Ayten, A., Tekke, M., & Agbaria, Q. (2019). On the links between positive religious coping, satisfaction with life and depressive symptoms among a multinational sample of Muslims. *International Journal of Psychology*, *54*(5), 678–686. https://doi.org/10.1002/ijop.12521

Ano, G. G., & Vasconcelles, E. B. (2005). Religious coping and psychological adjustment to stress: A meta-analysis. *Journal of Clinical Psychology*, *61*(4), 461–480. https://doi.org/10.1002/jclp.20049

Aten, J. D., Bennett, P. R., Hill, P. C., Davis, D., & Hook, J. N. (2012). Predictors of god concept and god control after hurricane Katrina. *Psychology of Religion and Spirituality*, *4*(3), 182–192. https://doi.org/10.1037/a0027541

Banu, H. (2020). *Adaptation and Preliminary Validation of the RCOPE for Muslims (RCOPE-M)* [Unpublished manuscript]. James Cook University, Singapore.

Bentzen, J. S. (2019). Why are some societies more religious than others? In J. P. Carvalho, S. Iyer, & J. Rubin (Eds.), *Advances in the economics of religion* (pp. 265–281). Palgrave Macmillan. https://doi.org/10.1007/978-3-319-98848-1_16

Best, M., Butow, P., & Olver, I. (2015). Do patients want doctors to talk about spirituality? A systematic literature review. *Patient Education and Counseling*, *98*(11), 1,320–1,328. https://doi.org/10.1016/j.pec.2015.04.017

Bhui, K., King, M. B., Dein, S., & O'Connor, W. (2008). Ethnicity and religious coping with mental distress. *Journal of Mental Health*, *17*(2), 141–151. https://doi.org/10.1080/09638230701498408

Brennan, E. (2014). *Religion in Southeast Asia: Diversity and the threat of extremes*. The Interpreter. https://www.lowyinstitute.org/the-interpreter/religion-southeast-asia-diversity-and-threat-extremes

de Zoysa, P., & Wickrama, T. (2011). Mental health and cultural religious coping of disabled veterans' in Sri Lanka. *Journal of Military and Veterans Health*, *19*(3), 4–12. https://search.informit.com.au/documentSummary;dn=681403054336260;res=IELHEA

Denworth, L. (2020). *How the COVID-19 Pandemic Could End*. Scientific American. https://www.scientificamerican.com/article/how-the-covid-19-pandemic-could-end1/

Faigin, C. A., Pargament, K. I., & Abu-Raiya, H. (2014). Spiritual struggles as a possible risk factor for addictive behaviors: An initial empirical investigation. *International Journal for the Psychology of Religion*, *24*(3), 201–214. https://doi.org/10.1080/10508619.2013.837661

Falb, M. D., & Pargament, K. I. (2013). Buddhist coping predicts psychological outcomes among end-of-life caregivers. *Psychology of Religion and Spirituality*, *5*(4), 252–262. https://doi.org/10.1037/a0032653

Falk, M. L. (2012). Gender, Buddhism and social resilience in the aftermath of the tsunami in Thailand. *South East Asia Research*, *20*(2), 175–190. https://doi.org/10.5367/sear.2012.0099

Fletcher, S. K. (2004). Religion and life meaning: Differentiating between religious beliefs and religious community in constructing life meaning. *Journal of Aging Studies*, *18*(2), 171–185. https://doi.org/10.1016/j.jaging.2004.01.005

French, D. C., Purwono, U., & Shen, M. (2020). Religiosity and positive religious coping as predictors of Indonesian Muslim adolescents' externalizing behavior and loneliness. *Psychology of Religion and Spirituality*. https://doi.org/10.1037/rel0000300

Gardner, T. M., Krägeloh, C. U., & Henning, M. A. (2014). Religious coping, stress, and quality of life of Muslim university students in New Zealand. *Mental Health, Religion & Culture*, *17*(4), 327–338. https://doi.org/10.1080/13674676.2013.804044

Ghorbani, N., Watson, P. J., Hajirasouliha, Z., & Chen, Z. J. (2016). Muslim distress mobilization hypothesis: Complex roles of islamic positive religious coping and punishing Allah reappraisal in Iranian students. *Mental Health, Religion and Culture*, *19*(6), 626–638. https://doi.org/10.1080/13674676.2016.1224824

Graham, J., & Haidt, J. (2010). Beyond beliefs: Religions bind individuals into moral communities. *Personality and Social Psychology Review*, *14*(1), 140–150. https://doi.org/10.1177/1088868309353415

Grover, S., Sarkar, S., Bhalla, A., Chakrabarti, S., & Avasthi, A. (2016). Religious coping among self-harm attempters brought to emergency setting in India. *Asian Journal of Psychiatry, 23*, 78–86. https://doi.org/10.1016/j.ajp.2016.07.009

Harrison, M. O., Koenig, H. G., Hays, J. C., Eme-Akwari, A. G., & Pargament, K. I. (2001). The epidemiology of religious coping: A review of recent literature. *International Review of Psychiatry, 13*(2), 86–93. https://doi.org/10.1080/09540260124356

Hassan, M., & Mehta, K. (2010). Grief experience of bereaved Malay/Muslim youths in Singapore: The spiritual dimension. *International Journal of Children's Spirituality, 15*(1), 45–57. https://doi.org/10.1080/13644360903565565

Ivtzan, I., Chan, C. P. L., Gardner, H. E., & Prashar, K. (2013). Linking religion and spirituality with psychological well-being: Examining self-actualisation, meaning in life, and personal growth initiative. *Journal of Religion and Health, 52*(3), 915–929. https://doi.org/10.1007/s10943-011-9540-2

Khan, Z. H., Watson, P. J., & Chen, Z. (2011). Differentiating religious coping from Islamic identification in patient and non-patient Pakistani Muslims. *Mental Health, Religion & Culture, 14*(10), 1,049–1,062. https://doi.org/10.1080/13674676.2010.550040

Khan, Z. H., Watson, P. J., & Chen, Z. (2012). Islamic religious coping, perceived stress, and mental well-being in Pakistanis. *Archive for the Psychology of Religion, 34*(2), 137–147. https://doi.org/10.1163/15736121-12341236

Khan, Z. H., Watson, P. J., & Chen, Z. (2016). Muslim spirituality, religious coping, and reactions to terrorism among Pakistani university students. *Journal of Religion and Health, 55*(6), 2,086–2,098. https://doi.org/10.1007/s10943-016-0263-2

Koenig, H. G., King, D. E., & Carson, V. B. (2012). *Handbook of Religion and Health* (2nd ed.). Oxford University Press.

Lau, G. P. W., & Ramsay, J. E. (2019). Salvation with fear and trembling? Scrupulous fears inconsistently mediate the relationship between religion and well-being. *Mental Health, Religion and Culture, 22*(8), 844–859. https://doi.org/10.1080/13674676.2019.1670629

Lazarus, R. S., & Folkman, S. (1984). *Stress, Appraisal, and Coping.* Springer Publishing Company.

Lee, S. A., Roberts, L. B., & Gibbons, J. A. (2013). When religion makes grief worse: Negative religious coping as associated with maladaptive emotional responding patterns. *Mental Health, Religion and Culture, 16*(3), 291–305. https://doi.org/10.1080/13674676.2012.659242

Lupfer, M. B., Tolliver, D., & Jackson, M. (1996). Explaining life-altering occurrences: A test of the "God-of-the-Gaps" hypothesis. *Journal for the Scientific Study of Religion, 35*(4), 379–391. https://doi.org/10.2307/1386413

Mayer, K. H., Bradford, J. B., Makadon, H. J., Stall, R., Goldhammer, H., & Landers, S. (2008). Sexual and gender minority health: What we know and what needs to be done. *American Journal of Public Health, 98*(6), 989–995. https://doi.org/10.2105/AJPH.2007.127811

Mohammadzadeh, A., & Najafi, M. (2018). The comparison of death anxiety, obsession, and depression between Muslim population with positive and negative religious coping. *Journal of Religion and Health, 59*, 1055–1064. https://doi.org/10.1007/s10943-018-0679-y

Neville, R. (2018). Philosophy of religion and the big questions. *Palgrave Communications, 4*(126). https://doi.org/10.1057/s41599-018-0182-9

Noh, H., Chang, E., Jang, Y., Lee, J. H., & Lee, S. M. (2016). Suppressor effects of positive and negative religious coping on academic burnout among Korean middle school students. *Journal of Religion and Health, 55*(1), 135–146. https://doi.org/10.1007/s10943-015-0007-8

Nurasikin, M. S., Khatijah, L. A., Aini, A., Ramli, M., Aida, S. A., Zainal, N. Z., & Ng, C. G. (2013). Religiousness, religious coping methods and distress level among psychiatric patients in Malaysia. *International Journal of Social Psychiatry, 59*(4), 332–338. https://doi.org/10.1177/0020764012437127

Pan, S. W., Tang, W., Cao, B., Ross, R., & Tucker, J. D. (2017). Buddhism and coping with HIV in China. *JANAC: Journal of the Association of Nurses in AIDS Care, 28*(5), 666–667. https://doi.org/ 10.1016/j.jana.2017.05.005

Pandey, J., & Singh, M. (2019). Positive religious coping as a mechanism for enhancing job satisfaction and reducing work-family conflict: A moderated mediation analysis. *Journal of Management, Spirituality and Religion, 16*(3), 314–338. https://doi.org/10.1080/14766086.2019.1596829

Pareek, M., Bangash, M. N., Pareek, N., Pan, D., Sze, S., Minhas, J. S., Hanif, W., & Khunti, K. (2020). Ethnicity and COVID-19 : An urgent public health research priority. *The Lancet, 395*(10234), 1,421–1,422. https://doi.org/10.1016/S0140-6736(20)30922-3

Pargament, K. I., Smith, B. W., Koenig, H. G., & Perez, L. (1998). Patterns of positive and negative religious coping with major life stressors. *Journal for the Scientific Study of Religion, 37*(4), 710–724. https://doi.org/10.2307/1388152

Pargament, K. I., Koenig, H. G., & Perez, L. M. (2000). The many methods of religious coping: Development and initial validation of the RCOPE. *Journal of Clinical Psychology, 56*(4), 519–543. https://doi.org/10.1002/(SICI)1097-4679(200004)56:4<519::AID-JCLP6>3.0.CO;2-1

Pearce, M. J., Pargament, K. I., Oxhandler, H. K., Vieten, C., & Wong, S. (2019). A novel training program for mental health providers in religious and spiritual competencies. *Spirituality in Clinical Practice, 6*(2), 73–82. https://doi.org/10.1037/scp0000195

Phillips, R. E., Cheng, C. M., Oemig, C., Hietbrink, L., & Vonnegut, E. (2012). Validation of a Buddhist coping measure among primarily non-Asian Buddhists in the United States. *Journal for the Scientific Study of Religion, 51*(1), 156–172. https://doi.org/10.1111/j.1468-5906.2012.01620.x

Pirutinsky, S., Rosmarin, D. H., & Pargament, K. I. (2009). Community attitudes towards culture-influenced mental illness: Scrupulosity vs. nonreligious OCD among orthodox jews. *Journal of Community Psychology*, *37*(8), 949–958. https://doi.org/10.1002/jcop.20341

Pung, R., Chiew, C. J., Young, B. E., Chin, S., Chen, M. I. C., Clapham, H. E., Cook, A. R., Maurer-Stroh, S., Toh, M. P. H. S., Poh, C., Low, M., Lum, J., Koh, V. T. J., Mak, T. M., Cui, L., Lin, R. V. T. P., Heng, D., Leo, Y. S., Lye, D. C., … Ang, L. W. (2020). Investigation of three clusters of COVID-19 in Singapore: Implications for surveillance and response measures. *The Lancet*, *395*(10229), 1,039–1,046. https://doi.org/10.1016/S0140-6736(20)30528-6

Quadri, S. A. (2020). COVID-19 and religious congregations: Implications for spread of novel pathogens. *International Journal of Infectious Diseases*, *96*, 219–221. https://doi.org/10.1016/j.ijid.2020.05.007

Ramsay, J. E., Tong, E. M. W., Chowdhury, A., & Ho, M. H. R. (2018). Teleological explanation and positive emotion serially mediate the effect of religion on well-being. *Journal of Personality*, *87*(3), 676–689. https://doi.org/10.1111/jopy.12425

Riggio, H. R., Uhalt, J., Matthies, B. K., Harvey, T., Lowden, N., & Umana, V. (2018). Explaining death by tornado: Religiosity and the god-serving bias. *Archive for the Psychology of Religion*, *40*(1), 32–59. https://doi.org/10.1163/15736121-12341349

Sibley, C. G., & Bulbulia, J. (2012). Faith after an Earthquake: A Longitudinal Study of religion and perceived health before and after the 2011 Christchurch New Zealand Earthquake. *PLoS ONE*, *7*(12). https://doi.org/10.1371/journal.pone.0049648

Silton, N. R., Flannelly, K. J., Galek, K., & Ellison, C. G. (2014). Beliefs about God and mental health among American adults. *Journal of Religion and Health*, *53*(5), 1,285–1,296. https://doi.org/10.1007/s10943-013-9712-3

Silva, P. De. (2006). The tsunami and its aftermath in Sri Lanka: Explorations of a Buddhist perspective. *International Review of Psychiatry*, *18*(3), 281–287. https://doi.org/10.1080/09540260600658270

Sinha, V. (2008). "Hinduism" and "Taoism" in Singapore: Seeing points of convergence. *Journal of Southeast Asian Studies*, *39*(1), 123–147. https://doi.org/10.1017/S0022463408000064

Steger, M. F., & Frazier, P. (2005). Meaning in life: One link in the chain from religiousness to well-being. *Journal of Counseling Psychology*, *52*(4), 574–582. https://doi.org/10.1037/0022-0167.52.4.574

Suthendran, S. (2017). *Perceived Preparedness in Working Therapeutically with Sexual and Gender Minorities: Perspectives of Trainee and Early-Career Clinical Psychologists in Singapore*. James Cook University, Singapore.

Tarakeshwar, N., Pargament, K. I., & Mahoney, A. (2003). Initial development of a measure of religious coping among Hindus. *Journal of Community Psychology, 31*(6), 607–628. https://doi.org/10.1002/jcop.10071

Thio, L.-A. (2009). Between Eden and Armageddon: Navigating "Religion" and "Politics" in Singapore. *Singapore Journal of Legal Studies*, 365–405. https://www.jstor.org/stable/24870523

Williams, J. A., Meltzer, D., Arora, V., Chung, G., & Curlin, F. A. (2011). Attention to inpatients' religious and spiritual concerns: Predictors and association with patient satisfaction. *Journal of General Internal Medicine, 26*(11), 1,265–1,271. https://doi.org/10.1007/s11606-011-1781-y

Xu, J. (2019). The lived experience of Buddhist-oriented religious coping in late life: Buddhism as a cognitive schema. *Journal of Health Psychology.* https://doi.org/10.1177/1359105319882741

Yao, H., Chen, J.-H., & Xu, Y.-F. (2020). Patients with mental health disorders in the COVID-19 epidemic. *The Lancet Psychiatry, 7*(4). https://doi.org/10.1016/S2215-0366(20)30090-0

Zinnbauer, B. J., & Pargament, K. I. (2000). Working with the sacred : Four approaches to religious and spiritual issues in counseling. *Journal of Counseling and Development, 78*(2), 162–171. https://doi.org/10.1002/j.1556-6676.2000.tb02574.x

# Chapter 8

# Supporting and Coping with Bereavement During and Post-Pandemic

Andy Hau Yan Ho, Oindrila Dutta,
Paul Victor Patinadan, and Geraldine Tan-Ho

## Introduction

The abrupt arrival of the new coronavirus in late-2019 has brought unprecedented chaos and loss to the world. According to the World Health Organisation (WHO), the number of confirmed cases of COVD-19 has reached more than 5.6 million by the fourth week of May, with over 353,000 deaths resulting from this highly infectious and fatal disease (WHO, 2020a). With no specific treatment currently available and the most optimistic date for a vaccine being at least 12 to 18 months away (Ghosh & Tan, 2020), social distancing will continue to play a dominant role in curbing the spread of infection, while fundamentally changing our way of life in a manner that could dislocate our relational bonds and social contracts. Particularly and most poignantly, a global pandemic like COVID-19 will profoundly transform the ways in which we face and cope with grief and bereavement.

Whether it is for sudden fatalities arising from the infectious disease or expected deaths owing to other chronic health conditions, we can no longer engage in the traditional customs and rituals that provide communal platforms of support that fully recognise the loss of life, acknowledge our

113

grief, and bring us comfort and solace in the face of mortality. Under a global pandemic where physical closeness and social intimacy are prohibited, carrying out last offices for or even bidding a final goodbye to our loved ones in their final days of life would not be possible. Such traumatic disruptions in our bereavement experience will have detrimental impacts in our post-loss adjustment and long-term recovery. This chapter will first examine the pain of disenfranchised grief with social distancing during COVID-19, discuss the critical need and evolving nature of bereavement customs and funerary rites during a pandemic, and finally explore how collective mourning and meaning reconstruction can aid in supporting and empowering bereavement recovery in a post-pandemic world.

## The Pain of Disenfranchised Grief and Social Distancing during COVID-19

Although every person will be touched by grief at some point in their lives, grieving the loss of a loved one during a pandemic can be a uniquely isolating and debilitating experience. Social distancing, while being one of the strongest measures to protect people through physical confinement, can greatly restrict interactions between individuals and their family members and friends who may be actively dying, prohibit any contact with the deceased body, reduce face-to-face connections between bereaved individuals and their support system of family and friends, as well as limit conventional rituals surrounding death and bereavement (Stieg, 2020).

In the wake of COVID-19, surviving family members and friends are unable to accompany their dying loved ones in hospitals in order to avoid the risks of infection; meanwhile others face challenges in hosting or attending memorial services with tight restrictions on physical gatherings and movement (Selman, 2020). Important ritualistic actions that play vital roles in publicly recognising the life of the deceased and formally acknowledging the loss of the mourners—meaningful goodbyes, imparting last words, congregating for funeral rites to bathe, pray, and watch over the dead body, as well as to share memories and stories of the deceased—have also been barred. Hence, bereaved individuals mourn not only the loss of their loved ones during a pandemic, but also the loss of significant rituals that legitimise and give meaning to their grief (Selman, 2020). Such complexity in the grieving process, as experienced "by those who incur a loss that is not, or cannot be, openly acknowledged, publicly mourned or socially supported", is termed "Disenfranchised Grief" (Doka, 1999, p. 37). Specifically, Doka explained that disenfranchised grief is a condition where the griever feels alone and isolated in their experience of loss, which makes it difficult to mourn and can further complicates grief reactions.

It is important to note here that during a pandemic, disenfranchised grief is not only unique to death-related losses, as the experience of grief can manifest from many different sources other than mortality. For instance, individuals may grieve multiple non-death losses during a prolonged virus outbreak that keeps them isolated; such as the loss of normalcy, social connections, intimate relationships, employment, financial income, education opportunities, certainties about the future, and a depreciating sense of personhood (Stieg, 2020). However, much of the ongoing dialogue in the media surrounding these experiences position them as indications of anxiety, depression, and mental health problems, instead of manifestations of loss (Kanter & Manbeck, 2020). This lack of acknowledgement or discussion of non-death losses would ultimately result in the disenfranchisement of grief (Gitterman & Knight, 2019). Moreover, when death-related losses are intertwined with non-death losses, with both not socially recognised by the larger community, individuals are denied the opportunity to express, work through, and receive support for their grief, increasing the potentiality of debilitating bereavement outcomes as well as complicated grief (Wallace *et al.*, 2020).

## The Taxonomic Perils of "Social" Distancing

In addition to the issue of disenfranchised grief which was described in the aforementioned section, individuals' mental well-being during a pandemic is further complicated by the taxonomy and meaning of the term "social distancing". Specifically, during a pandemic, it is essential to maintain safe physical distance between individuals to curb the spread of disease; however, the term "social distancing" implies that people can no longer fulfil their innate need to be relationally intimate, to connect with, and be comforted by others during difficult times, such as facing the death of a loved one or coping with non-death losses surrounding one's future (De Witte, 2020). Social distancing could also result in individuals who have lost a loved one to feel isolated more than ever, not just physically but relationally. As the word "social" contains relational implications, grieving individuals may feel that they are denied or should not expect the customary support that they would receive under normal circumstances. At the same time, families and friends may feel reluctant to offer their supportive presence under the connotation of relational separation. The term "social distancing" can thus create a mental bubble around pandemic survivors as they struggle to give and receive support throughout their grieving journeys.

In a step to emphasise the need for communal solidarity during COVID-19, the WHO revised its official language to replace the term "social distancing" with "physical distancing", as the latter holds the key to reducing the spread of disease (Anderson, 2020). By carefully selecting the most precise words to describe a public health measure, it is hoped that the reality of life amidst a pandemic can be accurately captured— where people are physically cocooned but socially connected through digital and other non-physical mediums (Perls, 2020). Experts also recommend that grievers could engage in meaningful online rituals to share their memories of who or what they have lost, and the impact that this has had on their life narrative (Stieg, 2020). For instance, by harnessing the power of social media, families and friends can share stories, prayers, and thoughts of the deceased through a Facebook post, in a group text, or during a video conference—all of which are plausible ways to offer a digital presence, a listening ear, and a shared sense of support to grieving persons. Furthermore, private and personalised rituals can be useful in acknowledging the realness of the loss while providing solace to those suffering from disenfranchised grief (Dutta *et al.*, 2020), and these may take the form of learning a food recipe in memory of the deceased (Patinadan *et al.*, 2020), or engaging in reflective journaling to document the life of the deceased to foster a healthy continuing bond (Ho *et al.*, 2020).

In the midst of a major lethal virus outbreak where losses abound and conventional grieving practices are overturned by the immediate and overwhelming need for public health and safety, rituals, especially those that are technology-enhanced, may well be one of the most effective tools to acknowledge, respect, and adequately mourn the realness of grief and loss that the community may not recognise or understand. The next section elaborates on the important role of such rituals in coping with grief during a global pandemic.

# Evolving Funerary and Bereavement Customs Amidst a Pandemic

Few events are as intrinsic to the human condition as bereavement rites and funerary rituals. Depending on the cultural context observed, these play varying parts of a dualistic role for both the deceased as well as living survivors. For the multi-religious belief systems present in Singapore, funerals furnish the deceased with the means for a successful migration to the afterlife; the ritualistic washing and shrouding for Muslims, the consecrated chanting for Buddhists, prayer and hymnals for Catholics and Christians, and the solemn conch call of the Hindus, among other similar practices (Bakar, 2016; Gatrad, 1994; Kiong, 2004). Survivors are presented with the opportunity for a public statement that their kin has died, and the larger community is afforded the response to sympathise and support. Pine (1995) posits four social functions of funerals present throughout history, with the event serving to:

1. Acknowledge and commemorate a death.
2. Provide a setting for body disposition.
3. Assist in reorienting the bereaved to their lives, which have been ruptured by death.
4. Demonstrate reciprocal economic and social obligations between the bereaved and their social world.

With the advent of COVID-19, however, a paradigm shift must occur in regard to how we practice these timeless functions. In early April 2020, the WHO provided a set of practical considerations for religious leaders and faith-based communities about safe burial practices; enunciating the conduct of "respectful and appropriate" funerals and comfort for mourners that minimise infection risk. Concerning ritual practice, it forwards modifications such as the use of Personal Protective Equipment (PPE) during washing and shrouding, for instance. Family members should be allowed to view the body, but follow local distancing restrictions, with no touching or kissing of the deceased, and thorough hand-washing is required post-viewing (WHO, 2020b). As physical distancing laws continue to tighten across the globe, streamlined funerals become harder to plan and perform, no doubt at the cost of significant socio-emotional distress for mourners. Open-casket viewings and the attendance of the larger community are effectively disavowed. Locally, the National Environment Agency (NEA) encourages a maximum of 10 family members in attendance at any one time, a disconsolate number when considered within the collective Asian perspective. For individuals who have died of COVID-19, their bodies are prepared for disposal within the hospital itself, being "double bagged and placed in a hermetically sealed coffin" (NEA, 2020). These restrictions are observed to conflict with the collective and symbolic responses to death usually endorsed to demonstrate the endurance of a society and its values (Yardley & Rolph, 2020).

Singapore sees an average of 1,700 deaths a month, and local funeral directors are observing a change in clientele requests; with an increased number of them shortening established rituals or forgoing wakes entirely (Tai, 2020). The insufficiency of contact with loved ones, coupled with the lack of after-death rituals make grieving during the pandemic doubly difficult (Ingravallo, 2020). Yardley and Rolph (2020) sound the clarion call to act now in the creation of new expressions of humanity (such as social death rituals) at this stage, positing that it may prevent harms to mental health and well-being associated with the complicated bereavement process that can follow a difficult death. Turning towards our working technological advancements may afford due dignity and compassion towards the deceased and the bereaved, and aid in the completion of several of Pine's (1995) social functions.

## Technology as a Recreative Medium

Perhaps no issue has been more cited (and vaguely explained) in recent literature as the use of technology during the COVID-19 pandemic. Hardware machinery and software programming options are often repurposed beyond their intended use as solutions to evolving concerns; new uses are being found for old tools, not without issues surfacing (Ting *et al.*, 2020). Live-stream funerals and wakes have become viable choices for extended family and community involvement during the funerary process (Hernandez & Berman, 2020). Though unfortunate that grief, once tactile and collective, has now dissipated into isolated experiences behind computer screens, the experience does allow a measure of continued connectivity. It is perhaps the unstructured nature of using existing technology in new ways, coupled with an unfamiliarity in navigating the social boundaries of funeral customs online, that must be addressed to effectively facilitate the evolved grieving process. Mourning rituals online, however, are not a novel phenomenon. As mentioned, popular social network sites such as Instagram and Facebook have options to memorialise pages for deceased loved ones, and there are also various paid e-obituary services available (van Ryn *et al.*, 2017). These options, however, are commemorative and static, with real-time interaction between mourners difficult.

The unforeseen, though perhaps not unexpected, ingenuity of the gaming community is one example of collective action for memorial in cyberspace. Elaborate funeral customs have been recorded in popular MMORPGs (Massively-Multiplayer Online Role-Playing Games) such as *World of Warcraft* and *Final Fantasy XIV*, where players adorn their avatars in sombre regalia at services to mourn the real-world passing of a guildsman and friend (Gibbs *et al.*, 2013; White, 2020). Players in farming simulator *Animal Crossing: New Horizons* have been observed to participate in memorial processions, and utilising the game's on-board design tools and pattern editor, are able to scan photos and customise monuments to their loved ones (Jones, 2020). Player-controlled avatars in these games are able to have conversations with each other at such events, sharing stories and exude a more tangible virtual presence than responses to a static page. They are even able to emote appropriately, with commands for crying, comforting, and laughing.

With regards to establishing the "new normal" of mourning and bereavement online, families are encouraged to create new rituals employing available technologies (Ohlheiser, 2020). These may include collated ideas on a Google document for memorial activities once restrictions have lifted, or videoconferencing for shared social events. Developers in the bereavement industry should also be encouraged to borrow from the creativity expressed by gamers; creating virtual worlds and platforms that host a suite of functionalities for continued and symbolic interaction. One example might be collective efforts from mourner-avatars adding towards the creation of a lasting e-monument on a platform. This can include resource-gathering tasks and crafting tasks seen in popular simulation games. *Minecraft*, for example, sees players collecting materials from the environment around them (such as wood from trees and stone from quarry rocks) to be used as construction materials for virtual architecture. Such activities serve as ultimate gateways to the recreation of meaning in the wake of bereavement.

# Meaning Reconstruction for Supporting Bereavement in a Post-Pandemic World

The many novel and technologically reinvented funerary and bereavement rituals that have emerged during the era of the new coronavirus underscore the vital importance of collective mourning, especially when communities are struck with large-scale sudden fatalities as well as expected mortality that cannot be properly acknowledged through traditional customs and practices. Such rituals not only serve to legitimise the grief experienced by those who have lost a loved one, they also provide a platform for remembrance and reflection on the life that was once lived by the deceased as well as the relationships that are shared with the bereaved. These rites of passage, traditional or virtual, are of utmost importance and necessity, for they involve the retelling of stories and reprocessing of narratives that help rebuild the assumptive worlds of grieving persons; worlds that have been shattered by deaths that are deemed unreal and non-sensical under a global pandemic.

As postulated by Janoff-Bulman (1992), the assumptive world is an organised cognitive schema—a set of fundamental beliefs and value system—that individuals hold dear, assume to be true when defining their own identity and self-worth, as well as for apprising the world and its events. These beliefs and values serve to ground and orientate people, providing them with a sense of reality, security, purpose, and meaning in life (Kauffman, 2002). In the event of a sudden and traumatic death or disenfranchised grief resulting from a pandemic, all of these beliefs and values which bring coherence and stability in a person's life are gravely challenged. As individuals fail to make sense of their loss, their assumptive worlds along with their fundamental beliefs and value system collapse, hope vanishes, and disillusionment emerges. In order to support the bereaved person to adapt and come to terms with a new reality without the deceased, a focus on making sense of the loss becomes paramount in the grieving process. The seminal work by Frankl (1992) contends that "the quest for meaning is the key to mental health and human flourishing", as meaning can empower individuals to overcome even the most tragic events.

Accordingly, it is essential for bereavement counselling and supportive programmes to provide a platform for grieving individuals to recreate their assumptive worlds and meaning structures in life, with the ultimate goal to restore their identity and purpose for living via a renewed and coherent sense of self (Neimeyer *et al.*, 2010). Central to this process is the griever's capacity to make sense of their loss through retelling the stories that situate the loss into their own life narrative (Neimeyer *et al.*, 2014). Such articulation and reintegration of past experiences with the perceived present and an imagined future through storytelling of one's life empower individuals to reconstruct their sense of meaning and identity amidst loss, grief and bereavement. This mechanism, known as narrative identity processing (Pals, 2006), has repeatedly been found to be a critical pathway for healing, healthy personality development, and positive self-transformation during adversities and difficult life experiences (McAdams, 2011). Furthermore, meaning reconstruction may result in benefit finding (Davis *et al.*, 1998), where individuals are able to see their loss within the larger global context of their lives, leading to the reprioritisation of goals, increased appreciation of life, improved relationship, and the prospect of post-traumatic growth (Tedeschi & Calhoun, 2004).

## The Caveat of Collective Grieving

While bereavement and mourning rituals are imperative for supporting grieving persons to make sense of and come to terms with their loss, many of these rites of passage occur collectively rather than individually during a pandemic. This is not surprising given the rhetoric that has headlined the political and social discussions of COVID-19; that the world is in this together, and so people should mourn together too. Indeed, the new coronavirus has left a trail of fatalities as well as economic, social, and political devastation throughout the globe in its wake, with no clear sign of stoppage. As such, people around the world grieve for an immeasurable amount of losses, one of the biggest that humanity has witnessed in the past century. This universally shared sense of loss has been labelled as "collective grief" by experts and media alike (Weir, 2020).

Yet, the recognition of such collective grief must not be used as a simplistic means in understanding and addressing the idiosyncratic nature of grief suffered by an individual who has lost their loved one in the midst of a pandemic. In fact, reducing one's unique and rich experience of loss to merely an occasion of communal mourning could very well further isolate the bereaved in their grief. This is because while collective grief is often unifying and widespread, it can also lack the depth and profundity of personal grief. After all, it is a very different experience to be grieving the hundreds of thousands of deaths of strangers as compared to grieving the single death of a beloved spouse.

Furthermore, deaths unrelated to COVID-19 are now either mentioned in passing or not at all. The collective grief and focus on the pandemic have been assimilated so strongly into our lives that the first question asked, whether or not aloud, when a death is announced, is "Was it caused by COVID-19?" Bereaved persons grieving the loss of a loved one who did not die from COVID-19 during this time may find support given hastily or briefly, sometimes made worse with the barriers of social distancing. In a world trying to survive a deadly new virus, deaths by familiar causes such as cancer or heart failure would not be given the attention or sentiment it once would have received. The caveat of collective grieving during COVID-19 is that while people as a community, nation, or world gather strength from such solidarity, people as bereaved spouses, parents, children, or friends could suddenly find themselves more alone in their grief than ever. Decades of seminal death studies and research have found that no matter the universality of death responses, grief remains a highly personalised journey (Doka, 2016). As such, practitioners and policymakers need to be mindful that while grief can be seen as a collective event during a global crisis, it is also a highly personal event during times of peril; people are indeed grieving together, but in immensely and profoundly different ways. In effect, interventions and supportive programmes must adopt and integrate both public health approaches that target the masses as well as personalised approaches that respect the idiosyncratic experiences of each grieving individual. Ultimately, the need to enhance grief literacy (Breen *et al.*, 2020), and push forth the movement of compassionate communities (Kellehear, 2005) is integral for facilitating and empowering bereavement recovery in a post-pandemic world.

## Conclusion

As the world grapples and comes to terms with a new post-pandemic normal where our way of life and social contracts will forever be changed, our innate need for human connections and intimacy following the loss of a loved one will remain immovable. Though COVID-19 has erected inaccessible boundaries, supportive bereavement and mourning, like a life well-lived, can transcend these physical limitations with due dignity, compassion, creativity and a little technological ingenuity.

# References

Anderson, J. (2020, April 3). Social distancing isn't the right language for what Covid-19 asks of us. *Quartz.* https://qz.com/1830347/social-distancing-isnt-the-right-language-for-what-covid-19-asks-of-us/

Bakar, S. H. B. A. (2016). *Betwixt and between: social marginalisation and ritual specialisation of Tamil Hindu undertakers in contemporary Singapore* (Doctoral dissertation, McGill University Montreal, Québec, Canada).

Breen, L. H., Kawashima, D., Joy, K., Cadell, S., Roth, D., Chow, A., & Macdonald, M. E. (2020). Grief literacy: A call to action for compassionate communities. *Death Studies.* https://doi.org/10.1080/07481187.2020.1739780

De Witte, M. (2020, March 19). Instead of social distancing, practice "distant socialising" instead, urges Stanford psychologist. *Stanford News.* https://news.stanford.edu/2020/03/19/try-distant-socializing-instead/

Doka, K. J. (1999). Disenfranchised grief. *Bereavement Care: For All those Who Help the Bereaved, 18*(3), 37–39. https://doi.org/10.1080/02682629908657467

Doka, K. J. (2016). *Grief is a journey: Finding your path through loss.* Simon & Schuster, Inc

Dutta, O., Tan-Ho, G., Choo, P. Y., Low C. X., Chong, P. H., Ng, C., Ganapathy, S., & Ho, A. H. Y. (2020). Trauma to transformation: The lived experience of bereaved parents of children with chronic life-threatening illnesses in Singapore. *BMC Palliative Care, 19*, 46. https://doi.org/10.1186/s12904-020-00555-8

Frankl, V. (1992). *Man's search for meaning.* 1946. Trans. Ilse Lasch.

Gatrad, A. R. (1994). Muslim customs surrounding death, bereavement, postmortem examinations, and organ transplants. *BMJ, 309*(6953), 521–523. https://doi.org/10.1136/bmj.309.6953.521

Gibbs, M. R., Carter, M., Arnold, M., & Nansen, B. (2013). Serenity now bombs a World of Warcraft funeral: Negotiating the morality, reality and taste of online gaming practices. *AoIR Selected Papers of Internet Research, 3.* https://journals.uic.edu/ojs/index.php/spir/article/view/8845

Ghosh, N., & Tan D. W. (2020, April 16). Record race to find Covid-19 vaccine cause for optimism. *The Straits Times.* https://www.straitstimes.com/world/united-states/record-race-to-find-covid-19-vaccine-cause-for-optimism

Gitterman, A., & Knight, C. (2019). Non-death loss: Grieving for the loss of familiar place and for precious time and associated opportunities. *Clinical Social Work Journal, 47*(2), 147–155. https://doi.org/10.1007/s10615-018-0682-5

Hernandez, A. R., & Berman, M. (2020, March 23). Grief amid the pandemic: Live-streamed funerals, canceled services and mourning left "unfinished". *The Washington Post*. https://www.stripes.com/news/us/grief-amid-the-pandemic-live-streamed-funerals-canceled-services-and-mourning-left-unfinished-1.623435

Ho, A. H. Y., Dutta, O., Tan-Ho, G., Tan, T. H. B., Low, C. X., Ganapathy S., Car, J., Ho, R. M. H., & Miao C. Y. (2020). A Novel Narrative e-Writing Intervention (NeW-I) of Children with Chronic Life-Threatening Illnesses: Protocol for an Open-Label Randomized Controlled Trial. *JMIR Research Protocol*. https://doi.org/10.21203/rs.2.12263/v1

Ingravallo, F. (2020). Death in the era of the COVID-19 pandemic. *The Lancet Public Health*, 5(5), e258. https://doi.org/10.1016/S2468-2667(20)30079-7

Janoff-Bulman, R. (1992). *Shattered assumptions*. Free Press.

Jones, C. (2020, April 14). How fans are using animal crossing: New horizons to remember lost loved ones. *ScreenRant*. https://screenrant.com/animal-crossing-new-horizons-fan-creations-memorial-funeral/

Kanter, J., & Manbeck, K. (2020, April 1). COVID-19 could lead to an epidemic of clinical depression, and the health care system isn't ready for that, either. *The Conversation*. http://theconversation.com/covid-19-could-lead-to-an-epidemic-of-clinical-depression-and-the-health-care-system-isnt-ready-for-that-either-134528

Kauffman, J. (2002). The psychology of disenfranchised grief: Liberation, shame, and self-disenfranchisement. In K. Doka (Ed.), *Disenfranchised grief: New directions, challenges, and strategies for practice* (pp. 61–77). Research Press.

Kellehear, A. (2005). *Compassionate cities: Public health and end-of-life care*. Routledge.

Kiong, T. C. (2004). *Chinese death rituals in Singapore*. Routledge.

McAdams, D. P. (2011) Narrative Identity. In S. Schwartz, K. Luyckx, and V. Vignoles (Eds.), *Handbook of Identity Theory and Research* (pp. 99–115). Springer.

National Environment Agency (2020). *COVID-19 circuit breaker measures: Frequently asked questions*. https://www.nea.gov.sg/our-services/public-cleanliness/environmental-cleaning-guidelines/circuit-breaker-measures/frequently-asked-questions

Neimeyer, R. A., Klass, D., & Dennis, M. R. (2014). A social constructionist account of grief: loss and the narration of meaning. *Death Studies*, 38(6–10), 485–498. https://doi.org/10.1080/07481187.2014.913454

Ohlheiser, A. (2020, April 13). The lonely reality of Zoom funerals. *MIT Technology Review*. https://www.technologyreview.com/2020/04/13/999348/covid-19-grief-zoom-funerals/

Pals, J. L. (2006). Narrative Identity processing of difficult life experiences: Pathways of personality development and positive self-transformation in adulthood. *Journal of Personality*, *74*(4), 1,079–1,100. https://doi.org/ 10.1111/j.1467-6494.2006.00403.x

Patinadan, P. V., Tan-Ho, G., Choo, P. Y., Tan-Ho, G., Low, X. C., & Ho, A. H. Y. (2020, April 27–May 2). *I Am What I Ate: The "Food for Life and Palliation" (FLiP) model for understanding the Lived Experience of nutritional assimilation among Singaporean Palliative Care Patients and their Families.* [Conference Presentation—Delayed to 2021 due to COVID-19]. 42nd Association for Death Education and Counseling Conference. Columbia, OI, United States.

Perls, T. (2020, March 20). *Social distancing: What it is and why it's the best tool we have to fight the coronavirus.* World Economic Forum. https://www. weforum.org/agenda/2020/03/social-distancing-coronavirus/

Pine, V. R. (1995). Funerals: Life's final ceremony. *A Challenge for Living: Dying, Death, and Bereavement*, *28*(2), 21–25. https://www.jstor.org/stable/26555300

Selman, L. (2020, April 17). How coronavirus has transformed the grieving process. *The Conversation.* http://theconversation.com/how-coronavirus-has-transformed-the-grieving-process-136368

Stieg, C. (2020, April 10). How to cope with grief during the COVID-19 pandemic. *CNBC.* https://www.cnbc.com/2020/04/10/how-to-cope-with-grief-during-the-covid-19-pandemic.html

Tai, J. (2020, April 26). Changing face of funerals amid Covid-19 circuit breaker rules. *The Straits Times.* https://www.straitstimes.com/singapore/changing-face-of-funerals

Tedeschi, R. G., & Calhoun, L. G. (2004). A clinical approach to posttraumatic growth. In P. A. Linley, & S. Joseph (Eds.), *Positive psychology in practice* (pp. 405–419). John Wiley & Sons, Inc.

Ting, D. S. W., Carin, L., Dzau, V., & Wong, T. Y. (2020). Digital technology and COVID-19. *Nature Medicine*, *26*(4), 459–461. https://doi.org/10.1038/ s41591-020-0824-5

van Ryn, L., Kohn, T., Nansen, B., Arnold, M., & Gibbs, M. (2017). Researching death online. In L. Hjorth, H. Horst, A. Galloway, & G. Bell (Eds.), *The Routledge companion to digital ethnography* (pp. 112–120). Routledge.

Wallace, C.L., Wladkowski, S.P., Gibson, A., & White, P. (2020). Grief during the COVID-19 pandemic: Considerations for palliative care providers. *Jounral of Pain and Symptom Management*, *60*(1), E70–E76. https://doi. org/10.1016/j.jpainsymman.2020.04.012

Weir, K. (2020, April 1). *Grief and COVID-19: Mourning our bygone lives.* American Psychological Association. https://www.apa.org/news/apa/2020/ 04/grief-covid-19

World Health Organization. (2020a). *WHO Coronavirus Disease (COVID-19) Dashboard.* https://covid19.who.int/

World Health Organization. (2020b). *Practical considerations and recommendations for religious leaders and faith-based communities in the context of COVID-19.* https://www.who.int/publications-detail/practical-considerations-and-recommendations-for-religious-leaders-and-faith-based-communities-in-the-context-of-covid-19

Yardley, S., & Rolph, M. (2020). Death and dying during the pandemic. *BMJ, 369,* m1472. https://doi.org/10.1136/bmj.m1472

# Section 3

# Digital Communication
# Related Issues

# Chapter 9

# The Role of Social Media During a Pandemic

Dymples Leong

## Introduction

The world has been battered by the novel coronavirus disease that emerged in 2019 (COVID-19). Countries are still grappling with the fallout and disruption caused by the global pandemic. Classified as a pandemic by the World Health Organisation [WHO], over 10 million confirmed cases were reported worldwide as of 3 July 2020 (Johns Hopkins University of Medicine, 2020). While public health experts have drawn parallels between COVID-19 and the 1918 influenza pandemic, previous pandemics had occurred in a different age—when access to media was limited and the advent of social media was yet inconceivable. Observers have noted that COVID-19 is a pandemic for the globalised, connected social media age.

The creation of social media platforms, such as Facebook, YouTube, and Twitter, has empowered individuals with direct informational access to global events. With engagement and dissemination capabilities, social media is seen as a necessity in our globalised, interconnected age. Social media has been effectively utilised to mobilise support for crisis and disaster response—videos, posts, and hashtags shared on social media on the 2019 Australian bushfires, for instance, drove home the message of ecological and economic damage on communities. Global expressions of solidarity and fundraising initiatives contributed to an increased global awareness of the bushfire crisis (Sokolov, 2020).

However, the duality of social media should not be ignored. Misinformation has the potential to disrupt effective responses to the crisis. Misinformation is further amplified by the fear and uncertainty triggered by the occurrence of a crisis, creating challenges to respond to such propagations in real-time. While efforts by technology companies and governments have contributed to tackling misinformation, it remains a persistent and perennial problem. This chapter examines the role of social media during a pandemic—its impact in responding to COVID-19, and its nature as a dynamic tool for resource and support mobilisation amplify the propensity for a misinformation "infodemic" to proliferate. Potential prescriptions and approaches in which social media can be leveraged during a pandemic are also explored.

## The Duality of Social Media

### An Influence on Public Response to the Pandemic

Social media has been a medium for multi-level responses towards tackling COVID-19. As countries enact lockdowns to restrict citizens' movements and tighten social distancing measures, social media has contributed towards connecting individuals, informing people about the news of COVID-19 developments, and also provided a form of escapism using entertainment content. Social media holds up a mirror to the physical world, fulfilling social interaction and information-seeking needs.

Social media is also utilised as a means to reinforce positive collective action. The expression of solidarity and support for frontline responders—medical practitioners, police, and other first responders—on social media inspired others to create community responses to spread awareness of the pandemic, and appreciation of healthcare professionals. Creative methods to get the message across have been utilised, including dance-inspired TikTok videos on handwashing and social distancing tips (Chiang, 2020). Community groups have organically sprung up, crowdsourcing valuable information and resources, with initiatives for dissemination to the wider community. In Singapore, Facebook was utilised for public resource mobilisation, ranging from providing students with tuition to the compilation of online grocery stores for home deliveries (Tan, 2020).

Ground-up initiatives supporting local hawkers have also emerged to support the food and beverage industry in Singapore, and collective action online was used by citizens to thank and encourage medical professionals for their service and care towards COVID-19 patients.

Individuals are not the only ones utilising social media frequently during the pandemic. Governments, public health institutions, and medical experts are communicating with the public directly through social media platforms as well (Leong, 2020a). Social media is widely seen as an essential crisis communication tool for governments and institutions. Crucial COVID-19 related information—ranging from lockdown regulations to available testing facilities—has been widely disseminated by local governments using social media. Social media groups, including Facebook groups, have been set up by various doctors and medical professionals to crowdsource COVID-19 information on social distancing, diagnosis, treatment, and other informational sources of medical assistance (Smith & Fay Cortez, 2020).

Public health experts have advocated that the provision of accurate information to the public is key to fighting the pandemic in this informational age. However, social media, while effective in pushing out information, can also hinder, or worse, undermine accurate information that could potentially help save lives.

### *"Infodemic" Challenge*

The WHO has termed the scale of COVID-19 related misinformation as an "infodemic"—specifically, the overabundance and proliferation of misinformation and rumours, making it difficult for the public to find trustworthy sources and reliable advice (United Nations, 2020). Misinformation on COVID-19 emerged in two periodic stages in 2020— from January to February, and from March to April. In the earlier days of COVID-19 in January to February, much was uncertain and unknown, including the origin and spread of the virus (Smith *et al.*, 2020). New developments and guidelines on public health regulations were updated daily on the internet and social media, resulting in occasional conflicting messages from public health authorities. Misinformation is subject to new discoveries and insights, and a mutable, evolving context makes misrepresentation harder to eliminate. COVID-19 misinformation, thriving on uncertainty, confusion, and fear, amplified the spread of supposed "cures" to combat the virus. The desire of individuals for answers and solutions provides fertile ground for the exploitation of susceptible audiences in engaging with misinformation.

The reverse of an information vacuum describes the later stage of COVID-19 from March onwards ("Covid-19 is spreading", 2020). As the virus spread to Europe and the United States, reporting of the virus increased exponentially, as global audiences attempted to seek understanding and clarity using social media platforms for individual and collective sense-making (Molla, 2020). Rapidly changing information and advice—mixed with the anxiety of the physical and emotional impacts of the virus—contributed to individuals feeling bewildered and overwhelmed by an overload of information. An information overload can potentially exacerbate a tendency towards selective exposure (Klausegger *et al.*, 2007). This filter bubble effect may strengthen confirmation bias and narrow the scope of information consumed.

Effective misinformation is often constructed with enough familiarity to be persuasive and is populated with descriptive language and vivid personal stories (Robson, 2020). This enables misinformation to drown out official information sources, further enabling its visibility on social media as such posts are often shared widely. Misinformation, which trends on social media, is often picked up by mainstream media with the intent of refuting fake news. However, while the intent is beneficent, this may backfire, inadvertently amplifying and reinforcing harmful messaging. This unintended backfiring, known as the Streisand effect, paradoxically brings more attention to the harmful messaging. Research has demonstrated that labelling information as disputed could lead social media users to believe unlabelled information as factual, even when it is revealed to be false (Pennycook *et al.*, 2019).

Bot-like behaviour on social media could also falsely drive content augmentation on social media, synthetically amplifying false emotional sentiment and discord (Ko, 2020). For instance, bot-like behaviour could create and amplify a false impression of grassroots debate regarding vaccine efficacy (Broniatowski *et al.*, 2018).

The unintended consequence of a social media connected world during a pandemic is the extent of misinformation which could undermine and undercut effective preventive and mitigative measures—measures which could help save lives. If misinformation is left unchecked, progress made by mitigation strategies and educational efforts on COVID-19 can be rapidly undone. Misinformation can amplify confusion, sow distrust, and could cause people to ignore public health guidelines and legislation, potentially endangering their lives and leading to disastrous consequences. For instance, rumours have resulted in the physical destruction of 5G property ("Mast fire probe", 2020), and the loss of lives due to hoaxes and premature evidence of alleged "cures" as effective remedies against COVID-19 ("Bootleg booze kills 27", 2020; Vigdor, 2020).

COVID-19-related rumours have also stirred up racial and xenophobic sentiment online. Existing prejudices against minorities and marginalised communities—the "othering" of minorities by majority communities—have been intensified due to the uncertainty and fear of the pandemic (Haynes, 2020). Islamophobic harassment and attacks in India had occurred when rumours of Muslims as vectors of COVID-19 began to spread on social media, heightening existing tensions between Hindu nationalists and the wider Muslim community in India (Regan *et al.*, 2020). In Singapore, racially-inflammatory posts on anti-Chinese sentiment were created on Twitter and shared widely online (Ho, 2020). In other parts of the world, including the United States, anxiety over coronavirus fears has contributed to acts of violence towards individuals of Asian descent (Ruiz *et al.*, 2020).

## Leveraging Social Media during a Pandemic

### *What have Technology Companies Done?*

COVID-19 is seen as a litmus test for social media companies in assessing their effectiveness against misinformation. Social media companies have understood the significance in which COVID-19 misinformation could be exploited, and have banded together to jointly tackle COVID-19 related misinformation (Statt, 2020). Facebook, for instance, has removed COVID-19 misinformation that is likely to contribute to "imminent physical harm", such as false claims about cures, or posts which could cause panic or unrest. Users who have interacted with such posts are notified, and are encouraged to engage with a WHO-managed Facebook page with accurate information on the virus (Rosen, 2020). Similarly, unverified claims by users on Twitter, such as incitement to social unrest or disorder, would be removed (Twitter, 2020). Going beyond tackling misinformation, Facebook automatically banned groups on its platform from mobilising anti-quarantine protests (Robertson, 2020).

Tech platforms are also making it easier for people to search for useful information on COVID-19. Google Search landing pages prominently feature resources from the WHO and country-specific health ministry advisories, as Google searches have soared since the pandemic broke. Searches have also unveiled prescient information relating to the categories of information people are searching for, and Google has made such information available for researchers and health officials to aid messaging efforts (Stephens-Davidowitz, 2020).

# Potential Prescriptions

While misinformation thrives on social media, strategies can be implemented to mitigate the misinformation in the midst of crisis situations. This section looks at potential prescriptions and approaches in which social media can be leveraged against misinformation during a pandemic.

## *Differentiated Messaging Strategies for Demographics*

While legislation such as Singapore's Protection from Online Falsehoods and Manipulation Act (POFMA) are effective in stemming the flow of COVID-19 misinformation, utilising non-legislative measures to push back against the potential impact of misinformation can be equally impactful. By understanding the pathways along which various demographics across the population commonly obtain information, communication practitioners can effectively push back against misinformation. While message delivery may vary according to different social media channels, the set of consistent facts must be at the crux of every messaging initiative. Demographic and social factors, including age, education, ethnicity, and language are important considerations when tailoring content messaging.

The emphasis on the positive usage of social media by tailoring messages for different audiences can be used to highlight the prominence of factual information. In Singapore, public engagement efforts through variety shows are livestreamed on Facebook, where celebrity and politician guests encourage the elderly to stay at home as much as possible (Sun, 2020). Engagement with younger demographics on social media is likewise crucial. Institutions, such as the WHO, have utilised multi-channel resources such as TikTok to better engage and inform young people (Leong, 2020b). This helps to ensure that myth-busting about COVID-19 reaches audiences in a way that they can understand and share with their community online.

Finding credible sources who can share public health messages can also be useful. Cultural groups often trust institutions they identify with, such as faith-based organisations. Religious leaders in various countries, for instance, advocated for practical ways to worship at home during the country's circuit breaker period.

## Highlighting Positive Social Norms Online

Positive social norms can also be reinforced by utilising differentiated messaging strategies for various demographics. Messaging containing positive social norms can be brought to greater visibility, and reduce the risk of bringing attention to harmful messaging.

Practitioners and policymakers can leverage on identifying and co-opting credible social media influencers to reinforce official COVID-19 guidelines issued by health authorities, by vetting and bringing on board familiar and credible individuals, and thereby enabling behavioural change to become highly salient and visible to selected audiences. Similar initiatives were undertaken by the Finnish government to combat the spread of misinformation. Selected social media influencers disseminated official COVID-19 information from the Finnish public health authorities. Fact-checkers ascertain the accuracy of content posted by influencers, and a handbook for influencers—for guidance on avoiding misinformation spread online—was published (United Nations Regional Information Centre for Western Europe, 2020). However, cultural contexts have to be taken into consideration. Different cultural and social norms and circumstances (e.g., perception levels of trust and credibility) exist for various countries, and practitioners should be mindful of limitations and resources in the co-option of influencers (Bavel *et al.*, 2020).

## Emphasise Information Utility in Messaging

Transparent, accurate, and actionable public health information, disseminated in a timely manner, is a powerful tool to tackle the COVID-19 pandemic. Information emphasising potential solutions to alleviate a problem is highly valued in a crisis situation. Information utility is defined as the extent to which information can aid individuals in making and evaluating decisions—the higher the individual perception of the practicality of a piece of information, the higher the willingness to engage with information (Knobloch-Westerwick & Kleinman, 2012). Content highlighting important information would be valued and ranked higher over other sources of information, leading to higher levels of audience engagement with the content online, as people prefer to share news with greater information utility (Berger & Milkman, 2012).[1] By highlighting the information utility of the message, communicators can assist audiences to cut through the information clutter in order to provide solutions to immediate problems.

Messaging issued by public health authorities and experts should specify steps needed to mitigate the pandemic. Simple bite-sized information, which seeks to allay concerns and fears, can serve to explain the situation as clearly as possible, while reducing technical jargon that contributes to providing actionable solutions that help citizens move forward (Mendy *et al.*, 2020). For instance, Singapore's Ministry of Health utilised visuals and explainer videos to educate the public on guidelines for staying safe during COVID-19 (Ministry of Health Singapore, 2020). Providing the public with tangible and actionable information will help alleviate stress, anxiety, and information fog (Starbird, 2020).

In order to increase the informational utility of a message, the various motivations of information search, and public opinion towards certain positions on health and policy should be uncovered. Mapping the public's motivations or drivers for information search can be used to address individuals' concerns towards relevant resources for assistance. Analysing common narratives online can enable the tailoring of adaptable messaging, and ensure nimble rebuttals of specific misinformation. The Center for Disease Control and Prevention (CDC) in the United States, for instance, noticed a spike in the number of online conversations centred on hydroxychloroquine, a drug that the Food and Drug Administration (FDA) has revoked for COVID-19 usage (U.S. Food & Drug Administration, 2020). Messaging warning the public against

---

[1]Information utility is also often found in the marketing strategies of global brands. Information utility marketing is used to provide a user with information that is useful, and therein lies the value proposition to the customer.

using unapproved drugs to treat COVID-19 was created in response, and was widely disseminated via traditional and social media channels.

## Raising the Prominence of Authoritative Sources of Information

Messages with high informational utility from credible sources should also be amplified across multiple channels. The ability of cross-sharing content on social media is an advantage, as different materials for varying demographics can be disseminated on multiple social media platforms. Target audiences who find such messages useful and practical are more likely to disseminate among their social networks by utilising social media platforms.

The visibility of authoritative sources of information should be emphasised during a pandemic. The challenge of differentiating between authoritative figures qualified to provide accurate information online, and influential figures who are not officially designated as authoritative sources on COVID-19, is becoming increasingly acute. Enlisting trusted voices can enable public health messages to be more effective in influencing behavioural change. Providing more exposure to public health experts can help minimise the "pull" of engaging with misinformation, as public health experts rank high as trusted and credible sources of information during a pandemic (Murray, 2020).

Public health experts should also build up their social media expertise. Understanding effective ways of presenting scientific research into simple, jargon-minimal messages or visual charts explaining findings of results can help the public better understand pandemic science. Experts can act as gatekeepers to assist in addressing misinformation and direct users to proper resources. Medical doctors on Instagram, for instance, can share relevant information on COVID-19 prevention using relatable examples in short video clips (Ohlheiser, 2020). Public health experts can also conduct livestream feeds of their experiences caring for COVID-19 patients, or post educational short videos for teenagers on TikTok. A trusted, credible expert providing prevention measures in a personal manner can lead to greater engagement and acceptance of behaviour change.

Social media companies can prominently feature social media posts or comments from authoritative public health experts on users' newsfeed or dashboards. This raised visibility allows users to know that there are credible resources, alongside official health ministries, to turn to for information and advice. Companies should also double down on efforts to weed out misinformation on their platforms.

### *Accuracy Nudge as Inoculation against Misinformation*

An accuracy nudge—a prompt to consider the accuracy of information on social media platforms—could hold promise in promoting critical thinking and discernment of factual accuracy before sharing online. Research from Pennycook *et al.* (2020) demonstrated that participants who were asked to rate the accuracy of a news headline in the contexts of both political and COVID-19-related misinformation were more discerning about the information they shared. Subtle nudges can help prime users to place information accuracy at their top-of-the-mind awareness, and be more aware of the potential consequences of sharing inaccurate information amongst social media networks.

Social media companies have enacted a similar nudge approach by displaying notifications when a user has interacted with COVID-19 misinformation which could cause imminent physical harm. Companies could potentially apply accuracy nudges to complement existing measures to mitigate engagement with misinformation. Accuracy nudges would be a subtle, content-neutral intervention. It could come in the form of automated reminders to provide a gentle nudge for users to question the veracity of information before sharing. As with all potential interventions, careful testing could enable companies to determine and refine reliable strategies for real-world application.

## Conclusion

As frontline responders do their best to develop a vaccine for the COVID-19 pandemic, efforts to inoculate the infodemic spread on social media should be conducted simultaneously. Misinformation can drown out the crux of the matter—the fact that accurate, scientific-backed information can and will help save lives. Mitigating strategies utilising social media as prescribed in this chapter can be leveraged against misinformation during a pandemic. If, and when the next pandemic arrives, the hope is for communicators and practitioners to be better prepared to utilise social media to communicate and effectively push back against misinformation online.

# References

Bavel, J.J.V., Baicker, K., Boggio, P.S., Capraro, V., … Willer, R. (2020). Using social and behavioural science to support COVID-19 pandemic response. *Nature Human Behaviour, 4*, 460–471. https://doi.org/10.1038/s41562-020-0884-z

Berger, J., & Milkman, K. L. (2012). What makes online content viral? *Journal of Marketing Research, 49*(2), 192–205. https://doi.org/10.1509/jmr.10.0353.

Bootleg booze kills 27 in Iran after coronavirus "cure" rumours. (2020). *The Straits Times.* https://www.straitstimes.com/world/middle-east/bootleg-booze-kills-27-in-iran-after-coronavirus-cure-rumours

Broniatowski, D., Jaminson, A., Qi, S., AlKulaib, L., Chen, T., Benton, A., Quinn, S., & Dredze, M. (2018). Weaponised health communication: Twitter bots and Russian trolls amplify the vaccine debate. *American Journal of Public Health, 108*(10), 1,378–1,384. https://doi.org/10.2105/AJPH.2018.304567

Chiang, A. [@austinchiangmd]. (2020). Coronavirus confusion pt. 2: surfaces. *TikTok.* https://www.tiktok.com/@austinchiangmd/video/6805277278726114565

Covid-19 is spreading rapidly in America. The country does not look ready. (2020). *The Economist.* https://www.economist.com/united-states/2020/03/12/covid-19-is-spreading-rapidly-in-america-the-country-does-not-look-ready

Haynes, S. (2020). As coronavirus spreads, so does xenophobia and anti-Asian racism. *TIME.* https://time.com/5797836/coronavirus-racism-stereotypes-attacks/

Ho, O. (2020). Action will be taken against Twitter user who made offensive posts to stoke racial tensions: Shanmugam. *The Straits Times.* https://www.straitstimes.com/singapore/action-will-be-taken-against-twitter-user-who-made-offensive-posts-to-stoke-racial

Johns Hopkins University of Medicine. (2020). *Coronavirus dashboard by the centre for system science and engineering.* https://coronavirus.jhu.edu/map.html

Klausegger, C., Sinkovics, R., & Zou, H. (2007). Information overload: A cross-national investigation of influence factors and effects. *Marketing Intelligence & Planning, 25*(7). https://doi.org/10.1108/02634500710834179

Knobloch-Westerwick, S., & Kleinman, S. (2012). Preelection selective exposure: Confirmation bias versus informational utility. *Communication Research, 39*(2), 170–193. https://doi.org/10.1177/0093650211400597

Ko, R. (2020). Meet "Sara", "Sharon" and "Mel": why people spreading coronavirus anxiety on Twitter might actually be bots. *The Conversation.* https://theconversation.com/meet-sara-sharon-and-mel-why-people-spreading-coronavirus-anxiety-on-twitter-might-actually-be-bots-134802

Leong, D. (2020a). Commentary: Telegram, the Powerful COVID-19 Choice of Communications by Many Governments. *Channel News Asia.* https://www. channelnewsasia.com/news/commentary/coronavirus-covid-19-government-telegram-whatsapp-fake-news-info-12707902

Leong, D. (2020b). Battling COVID-19, One TikTok Challenge at a Time. *The Diplomat.* https://thediplomat.com/2020/03/battling-covid-19-one-tiktok-challenge-at-a-time/

Mast Fire Probe Amid 5G Coronavirus Claims. (2020). *British Broadcasting Corporation.* https://www.bbc.com/news/uk-england-52164358

Mendy, A., Stewart, M., & VanAkin, K. (2020). A leader's guide: Communicating with teams, stakeholders, and communities during COVID-19. *McKinsey & Company.* https://www.mckinsey.com/business-functions/organization/our-insights/a-leaders-guide-communicating-with-teams-stakeholders-and-communities-during-covid-19#

Ministry of Health Singapore. (2020). *Content you can use.* https://www.moh. gov.sg/covid-19/resources

Molla, R. (2020). How coronavirus took over social media. *Recode.* https://www. vox.com/recode/2020/3/12/21175570/coronavirus-covid-19-social-media-twitter-facebook-google

Murray, M. (2020). In new poll, 60 percent support keeping stay-at-home restrictions to fight coronavirus. *NBC.* https://www.nbcnews.com/politics/meet-the-press/poll-six-10-support-keeping-stay-home-restrictions-fight-coronavirus-n1187011

Ohlheiser, A. (2020). Doctors are now social-media influencers. They aren't all ready for it. *MIT Technology Review.* https://www.technologyreview.com/2020/04/26/1000602/covid-coronavirus-doctors-tiktok-youtube-misinformation-pandemic/

Pennycook, G., Bear, A., Collins, E., & Rand, D. (2019). The implied truth effect: Attaching warnings to a subset of fake news headlines increases perceived accuracy of headlines without warnings. *Management Science.* https://doi. org/10.1287/mnsc.2019.3478

Pennycook, G., McPhetres, J., Zhang, Y., & Rand, D. (2020). Fighting COVID-19 misinformation on social media: Experimental evidence for a scalable accuracy nudge intervention. *Psychological Science.* https://doi.org/10.31234/osf.io/uhbk9

Regan, H., Sur, P., & Sud, V. (2020). India's Muslims feel targeted by rumors they're spreading Covid-19. *CNN.* https://edition.cnn.com/2020/04/23/asia/india-coronavirus-muslim-targeted-intl-hnk/index.html

Robson, D. (2020). Why smart people believe coronavirus myths. *BBC Future.* https://www.bbc.com/future/article/20200406-why-smart-people-believe-coronavirus-myths

Robertson, A. (2020). Facebook is banning protest events that violate social distancing rules. *The Verge.* https://www.theverge.com/2020/4/20/21228036/facebook-ban-event-protest-misinformation-government-social-distancing

Rosen, G. (2020). An Update on Our Work to Keep People Informed and Limit Misinformation About COVID-19. *Facebook.* https://about.fb.com/news/2020/04/covid-19-misinfo-update/

Ruiz, N.G., Horowitz, J.M., & Tamir, C. (2020). Many Black and Asian Americans say they have experienced discrimination amid the COVID-19 outbreak. *Pew Research Center.* https://www.pewsocialtrends.org/2020/07/01/many-black-and-asian-americans-say-they-have-experienced-discrimination-amid-the-covid-19-outbreak/

Smith, M., & Fay Cortez, M. (2020). Doctors turn to social media to develop Covid-19 treatments in real time. *Bloomberg.* https://www.bloomberg.com/news/articles/2020-03-24/covid-19-mysteries-yield-to-doctors-new-weapon-crowd-sourcing

Smith, M., McAweeney, E., & Ronzaud, L. (2020). The COVID-19 "Infodemic". *Graphika.* https://public-assets.graphika.com/reports/Graphika_Report_Covid19_Infodemic.pdf

Sokolov, M. (2020). Social media as a force for good: the case of Australian bushfires. *The Drum.* https://www.thedrum.com/opinion/2020/02/17/social-media-force-good-the-case-australian-bushfires

Starbird, K. (2020). How a crisis researcher makes sense of Covid-19 misinformation. *Medium.* https://onezero.medium.com/reflecting-on-the-covid-19-infodemic-as-a-crisis-informatics-researcher-ce0656fa4d0a

Statt, N. (2020). Major tech platforms say they're "jointly combating fraud and misinformation" about COVID-19. *The Verge.* https://www.theverge.com/2020/3/16/21182726/coronavirus-covid-19-facebook-google-twitter-youtube-joint-effort-misinformation-fraud

Stephens-Davidowitz, S. (2020). Google searches can help us find emerging Covid-19 outbreaks. *The New York Times.* https://www.nytimes.com/2020/04/05/opinion/coronavirus-google-searches.html

Sun, D. (2020). E-getai entertains the elderly at home. *The New Paper.* https://www.tnp.sg/news/singapore/e-getai-entertains-elderly-home

Tan, A. (2020). COVID-19: Hope for S'pore hawkers comes in the form of a booming Facebook community. *Vulcan Post.* https://vulcanpost.com/696286/hawkers-united-facebook-group-singapore/

Twitter. (2020). *Coronavirus: Staying safe and informed on Twitter.* https://blog.twitter.com/en_us/topics/company/2020/covid-19.html#unverifiedclaims

United Nations. Department of Global Communications. (2020). *UN tackles "infodemic" of misinformation and cybercrime in COVID-19 crisis.* https://www.un.org/en/un-coronavirus-communications-team/un-tackling-%E2%80%98infodemic%E2%80%99-misinformation-and-cybercrime-covid-19

United Nations Regional Information Centre for Western Europe. (2020). *COVID-19: The power of the hashtag.* https://unric.org/en/covid-19-the-power-of-the-hashtag/

U.S. Food & Drug Administration. (2020). *FDA cautions against use of hydroxychloroquine or chloroquine for COVID-19 outside of the hospital setting or a clinical trial due to risk of heart rhythm problems.* https://www.fda.gov/drugs/drug-safety-and-availability/fda-cautions-against-use-hydroxychloroquine-or-chloroquine-covid-19-outside-hospital-setting-or

Vigdor, N. (2020). Man fatally poisons himself while self-medicating for Coronavirus, doctor says. *New York Times.* https://www.nytimes.com/2020/03/24/us/chloroquine-poisoning-coronavirus.html?smtyp=cur&smid=fbnytimes&fbclid=IwAR3DvxiVrr_BbgGNqAmptMLC8RhiW4btzE4ruCRznkFYpj-oLIqtI8ELpxk&fbclid=IwAR2wultjKE4yzoHKKGynjmy-ODslfV7DIzF8surA5ZkpHDP0rKVPz2SFwUI

Chapter 10

# Managing the Spread of Misinformation During COVID-19

Xingyu Ken Chen

## Introduction

Around the world, misinformation and rumours began spreading in tandem with the COVID-19 outbreak. From speculations about the virus turning people into zombies ("Coronavirus Won't Turn", 2020) to dubious advice about using alcohol ("Alcohol Does Not", 2020) or cigarettes ("Misleading Information", 2020) to ward off the virus, much of such misinformation and rumours are driven by fear, which can prove as contagious as the virus.

During such a time of uncertainty where there is a deluge of misinformation on COVID-19 and fears arising over how the virus is transmitted, it is important for the public to remain alert and turn to official sources of information on the outbreak. Additionally, public service officers should also be on guard against falling to or spreading misinformation. Public service officers are not immune to falling prey to misinformation, but given their roles and responsibilities in maintaining public order and calm during this period, they should be more vigilant against misinformation.

The spread of misinformation during an outbreak can have serious consequences on a society's collective resilience, ranging from social disharmony to panic buying. Due to the Chinese origin of the virus, it accentuated a racist, xenophobic streak in some people (Kok, 2020).

Locally, Abdul Halim Abdul Karim, a religious teacher, made a Facebook post claiming that the virus was divine retribution for China's treatment of the Muslim Uighurs and that the Chinese caused the virus to spread as they were less hygienic as compared to Muslims ("MHA to Look Into", 2020). Such comments are highly misleading about the nature of the outbreak and are troubling, given that they perpetuate negative sentiments towards a particular group of people.

Additionally, the government issued multiple correction notices relating to the misinformation surrounding the virus as the misinformation could spark public panic. One correction notice was directed against a *States Times Review* article which claimed that face masks had run out ("Correction Directions Issued", 2020). Another correction notice was issued against a HardwareZone forum post which claimed that someone had died from the virus on 26 January 2020 ("SPH Magazines Complies", 2020). As the COVID-19 outbreak continues, it is unlikely that misinformation or the fear related to the COVID-19 would stop. In fact, the fear surrounding the virus should be understood in order to develop evidence-based strategies to manage the spread of fear and misinformation.

## How Fear Drives the Spread of Misinformation during an Outbreak

The spread of disease is often coupled with the spread of misinformation and fear (Epstein *et al.*, 2008), and this has been seen in multiple outbreaks in the past. For example, during the Ebola outbreak in Nigeria, people were known to consume large quantities of saltwater due to the misinformation that saltwater could fend off Ebola (Bali *et al.*, 2016). Similarly, during the Severe Acute Respiratory Syndrome (SARS) outbreak, the Chinese public began killing thousands of pets, including dogs and cats that they feared were carrying the SARS virus (Bowen & Heath, 2007). However, these actions had no effect on containing either outbreaks, and in some cases, accelerated the spread of the disease.

### *Over-trusting Any Warnings Due to Fear*

There are few explanations for why people are over-trusting of information (including misinformation) about an outbreak. In general, people tend to be more trusting of information regarding dangers (Fessler *et al.*, 2014). From a functional perspective, being more trusting of information regarding dangers is a helpful survival strategy for individuals and groups. At the individual level, fearful individuals are more likely to pay attention to information about their surroundings so that they can detect, prevent, or escape from danger (Sehlmeyer *et al.*, 2009). At the group level, fearmongering is more likely to receive attention and be passed on, as this is a process which can quickly signal to the entire group that there is a danger that they need to attend to (Kelly *et al.*, 2016). As a result, these groups are more likely to survive threats in their environment when they pay attention to such information that is being spread by fearmongering.

Over-trusting information on dangers is likely to enable the unhindered spread of information (regardless of its veracity) as it is driven by fear and a desire to survive. Moreover, this bias in people is particularly salient during crises as people are more likely to seek information about what they can do to protect themselves during a crisis (Lundgren & McMakin, 2013), making them more vulnerable to misinformation.

## Social Media Amplifies the Spread of Misinformation and Fear

The issue is worsened when people take to social media to share information about COVID-19. As compared to SARS, the challenge posed by misinformation has drastically increased given advancements in information technology—i.e., social media (Lim, 2020). Recent studies have shown that during recent outbreaks of diseases such as Middle East Respiratory Syndrome (MERS), social media has become a popular method for individuals to communicate and obtain relevant information (Choi *et al.*, 2017; Yoo *et al.*, 2016). However, not all information is helpful or accurate, as evidenced by the flood of misinformation in prior outbreaks such as Ebola (Bali *et al.*, 2016).

In the past, misinformation was more manageable as traditional news outlets could be held responsible for the dissemination and verification of information. News outlets were the primary source of information for people when they sought information about diseases or crises. Government agencies would partner with national television networks and newspapers to disseminate information about disease prevention measures (Ho *et al.*, 2013; Tay *et al.*, 2010). Even if people speculated about the aspects of the crises within their own social groups, the speculation remains localised.

The widespread usage of social media meant that a large number of people are receiving information from a disparate number of sources, such as social media or messaging platforms (Newman *et al.*, 2019). For the case of COVID-19 in Singapore, Chua (2020a, 2020b) identified spikes in sharing of news on Facebook during the announcement of the first infected patient and the announcement of DORSCON Orange.

The democratisation of content publishing brought about by social media also contributed to an exponential jump in the number of people who can produce and disseminate information. However, the same democratisation of content publishing has also exacerbated the problem of misinformation. This is because not all authors go through the rigour of checking the accuracy of their content before publishing. In addition, there is a perceived lack of consequences for publishing misinformation, given the relative invisibility and safety, which the internet offers to its users (Dredze *et al.*, 2016; Ghenai & Mejova, 2018). It is possible that the perceptions of invisibility and safety from being anonymous online means that people may feel that there are fewer consequences for their actions (e.g., being identified or shamed), and thus they may feel less inhibited in sharing misinformation.

Prior research found that during outbreaks, information that is shared by users on social media also tend to contain more misinformation (see Oyeyemi *et al.*, 2014; Vijaykumar *et al.*, 2018). This can create a vicious cycle where a surge in misinformation—which can incite more fear in the public—drives more misinformation that is being shared out of fear. In Singapore, unofficial channels of information have sprung up in response to the COVID-19 outbreak, where people could discuss and share information about the crisis. Chen and Neo (2020) identified several types of misinformation being propagated on Telegram chats in Singapore, such as fake information about the virus, conspiracy theories about COVID-19, as well as pseudo-scientific advice about how to fight off the coronavirus.

By design, social media is set up to amplify content based on popularity and relevance for its user (Barnhart, 2019). Hence, misinformation about an outbreak tends to go viral on social media, given people's innate sensitivity to information regarding dangers (as highlighted earlier). In fact, misinformation about cures for the virus and false warnings are abundant on social media (Thomas, 2020), as they can easily find an audience among people who are worried or fearful.

## Secondary Effects of Fear and Misinformation on Collective Resilience

The combination of fear and misinformation can lead to behaviours that can undermine the collective resilience of a society during an outbreak. The public could delay seeking medical treatment due to misinformation on appropriate means of treatment. Similarly, misinformation about shortages of certain items such as toilet paper and basic food items can and have led to panic buying (Taylor, 2020). This has certainly been seen in many countries around the world, such as the United States, New Zealand, Malaysia, and even Singapore (Lufkin, 2020). Such actions leave a society worse off than before as it diverts resources away from where it is needed during a pandemic.

Misinformation can also undermine collective resilience of a society by exacerbating other kinds of negative social effects such as increasing xenophobic sentiments. For example, some netizens were quick to attribute the cause of the outbreak to the eating habits of the Chinese, especially in light of a video showing a Chinese woman consuming bat soup. However, this attribution turned out to be misleading as the video was shot in Palau—a country located in the western Pacific Ocean, not China—and was made years before the COVID-19 outbreak (Kok, 2020).

# How to Avoid Falling Prey to Misinformation

The following section outlines five tips for individuals to avoid falling prey to misinformation during this time of fear and uncertainty posed by the ongoing COVID-19 situation.

## Seek Updates on the Virus from Reliable Channels of Information

Due to the deluge of misinformation online, one way to avoid falling prey to it is to consult reliable sources of information. Some methods such as relying on one's intuition or turning to one's social network to get accurate information about the virus can be unreliable, but they are frequently used. For example, Tandoc *et al.* (2018) identified that people tended to rely on their own judgment to identify if a piece of information is accurate or not. If it was insufficient, they would then rely on external sources such as their family and friends, or institutional sources—e.g., news from the media or fact-checking sites (Tandoc *et al.*, 2018). In Singapore, there are a few sources of interest where the public can get reliable information about the coronavirus situation. For example, in response to the COVID-19 outbreak, there is the gov.sg WhatsApp channel which the public can sign up to receive updates about the virus, as well as the Ministry of Health's website (Gov.sg, 2020).

## *Practice Emotional Scepticism when Feeling Afraid*

Although people are hardwired to respond to fear, it does not mean that individuals are helpless against fear. One thing people can do is to cultivate emotional scepticism as a form of defence against misinformation (Chen, 2019; "The rise and fall of", 2017). Emotional scepticism describes a mindset where people should be highly cautious when they experience strong emotional impulses as they could be easily influenced and manipulated by external factors. One simple way to avoid making rash decisions (e.g., sharing unverified information) out of fear is to wait until one feels calm. Research indicates that a "down-time" of between 10 to 60 minutes (Gneezy & Imas, 2014; Verduyn *et al.*, 2009) can help to reduce the effect and intensity of emotions experienced by an individual.

## *Be Vigilant Online by Exercising a Healthy Dose of Scepticism*

A healthy dose of scepticism is needed when individuals are navigating information online (Wineburg & McGrew, 2017). Information on the internet is not always what it seems—even screenshots claiming to show articles from respectable outlets can be faked ("CNA Debunks Fake Tweet", 2020). Hence, one important practice is to always verify that the information one accepts is accurate. This is important as a healthy level of scepticism can help to counter the effects of misinformation in individuals (Lewandowsky *et al.*, 2012), as they are primed to expect misinformation and hence will be on the lookout for it.

One thing individuals can do is to check if fact-checking sites (e.g., AFP Singapore Fact Check, Factually, Black Dot Research) have debunked the claim, or if the story is being reported by multiple reputable news outlets (Kiely & Robertson, 2016). One good rule of thumb is that individuals should check the veracity of the information if the information has no links to an official source about the pandemic (Caulfield, 2017). There are some fact-checkers in Singapore who can perform credible fact-checking for misinformation and post the findings on their websites. For example, Facebook, in partnership with Agence France-Presse (a recognised signatory by the International Fact-Checking Network), has been fact-checking fake news found in Singapore across several languages such as English, Mandarin, and Malay (Kwang, 2019).

## *Do Something, Rather than Nothing Against the Spread of Misinformation*

Even in instances when people do not fall for misinformation, research indicates that they would ignore misinformation when they encounter it (Tandoc, 2017), or not share it with others (Tan *et al.*, 2019). However, during an outbreak when there is communal fear and widespread misinformation, there is a need for collective efforts to counter misinformation proactively. Actions, such as reporting the misinformation or publicly sharing debunked information, can mitigate the risk of others falling for it. The community should be encouraged to take a screenshot of dubious content encountered and then forward it to news agencies or fact-checkers (Funke, 2018). This would prevent more people from falling for misinformation, as the fact-checkers and news agencies are able to follow up on the misinformation, and if necessary, disseminate debunked information to a wider audience.

## *Affirm Good Intentions when Countering Misinformation from Friends and Family*

People often worry about harming relationships with friends and family members when they correct them for sharing misinformation (Dixit, 2017; Silverman, 2019). To overcome this, a three-step approach can be adopted. First, understand where the other person is coming from (Silverman, 2019). This is done by monitoring one's tone of voice by keeping it soothing, rather than confrontational and avoid voicing denials and disagreements first (Voss & Raz, 2016). It does not mean that individuals should not disagree with the other party. Instead, they should suspend their disagreements first so that they can hear out the other person.

Second, help the other person feel heard. This is done by acknowledging the validity of the other person's emotions (Voss & Raz, 2016) and good intentions (Lewandowsky *et al.*, 2012). When people feel heard, it reduces the frustration and ill-will they experience and makes them less hostile to towards the third step. Thirdly, debunk the misinformation and directing them to relevant, trusted sources for verified information. Evidence suggests that merely stating that the misinformation is inaccurate is not enough, as there is a gap in their understanding that needs to be filled with accurate information so that they will not continue believing the misinformation (Cook & Lewandowsky, 2011).

## Conclusion

Given that the spread of disease, such as COVID-19, is often coupled with the spread of misinformation and fear, understanding how fear drives the spread of misinformation is a key aspect to fighting it. This chapter looked at a few ways to fight misinformation during such situations: (1) seek information from reliable sources, (2) practice emotional scepticism, (3) be vigilant in checking information online, (4) do something, rather than nothing in order to counter misinformation, and (5) affirm good intentions when misinformation is from one's family and friends.

## Acknowledgement

The views expressed in this chapter are the author's only and do not represent the official position or view of the Ministry of Home Affairs, Singapore.

## References

Alcohol does not protect against COVID-19; access should be restricted during lockdown. (2020, April 14). *World Health Organisation.* https://www.euro. who.int/en/health-topics/health-emergencies/coronavirus-covid-19/news/ news/2020/4/alcohol-does-not-protect-against-covid-19-access-should-be-restricted-during-lockdown

Bali, S., Stewart, K. A., & Pate, M. A. (2016). Long shadow of fear in an epidemic: Fearonomic effects of Ebola on the private sector in Nigeria. *British Medical Journal Global Health, 1*(3). https://doi.org/10.1136/bmjgh-2016-000111

Barnhart, B. (2019, August 13). *Everything you need to know about social media algorithms*. Sprout Social. https://sproutsocial.com/insights/social-media-algorithms/

Bowen, S. A., & Heath, R. L. (2007). Narratives of the SARS epidemic and ethical implications for public health crises. *International Journal of Strategic Communication, 1*(2), 73–91. https://doi.org/10.1080/15531180-701298791

Caulfield, M. (2017). *Web literacy for student fact-checkers*. Pressbooks.

Chen, X. K. (2019). Fake news after a terror attack: Psychological vulnerabilities exploited by fake news creators. In M. Khader, L. S. Neo, D. D. Cheong, & J. Chin (Eds.), *Learning from Violent Extremist Attacks: Behavioural Sciences Insights for practitioners and policymakers* (pp. 435–451). World Scientific Press.

Chen, X. K., & Neo, L. S. (2020). What are the topics discussed by the Singaporean public on about COVID-19? An exploratory analysis of telegram chats. *SSRN.* https://doi.org/10.2139/ssrn.3608579

Choi, D-H., Yoo, W., Noh, G-Y., & Park, K. (2017). The impact of social media on risk perceptions during the MERS outbreak in South Korea. *Computers in Human Behavior, 72*, 422–431. https://doi.org/10.1016/j.chb.2017.03.004

Chua, C. H. (2020a, January 31). *Going Viral: How Singaporeans Reacted On FB As Wuhan Coronavirus Outbreak Worsened*. Analytix Labs. https://www.analytix-labs.com/insights/wuhan

Chua, C. H. (2020b, February 14). *Behind The Panic Buying: A Surge On FB As S'pore Raised Its Virus Alert Level*. Analytix Labs. https://www.analytix-labs.com/insights/panic-buying

CNA debunks fake tweet announcing school closure due to coronavirus outbreak. (2020, February 7). *Channel NewsAsia.* https://www.channelnewsasia.com/news/singapore/cna-debunks-fake-tweet-announcing-school-closure-due-to-12404934

Cook, J., & Lewandowsky, S. (2011). *The Debunking Handbook*. University of Queensland.

Coronavirus won't turn you into a zombie, Malaysia says. (2020, February 2). *South China Morning Post.* https://www.scmp.com/news/asia/southeast-asia/article/3048599/coronavirus-wont-turn-you-zombie-malaysia-says

Correction directions issued over claims of Singaporeans contracting Wuhan coronavirus, shortage of masks. (2020, January 31). *Channel NewsAsia.* https://www.channelnewsasia.com/news/singapore/wuhan-virus-pofma-direction-article-facebook-12372632

Dixit, P. (2017, December 20). Older Indians Drive Millennials Crazy On WhatsApp. This Is Why They're Obsessed. *BuzzFeed News.* https://www.buzzfeednews.com/article/pranavdixit/older-indians-drive-millennials-crazy-on-whatsapp-this-is

Dredze, M., Broniatowski, D. A., & Hilyard, K. M. (2016). Zika vaccine misconceptions: A social media analysis. *Vaccine, 34*(30), 3,441–3,442. https://doi.org/10.1016/j.vaccine.2016.05.008

Epstein, J. M., Parker, J., Cummings, D., & Hammond, R. A. (2008). Coupled contagion dynamics of fear and disease: Mathematical and computational explorations. *PLoS ONE, 3*(12). https://doi.org/10.1371/journal.pone.0003955

Fessler, D. M. T., Pisor, A. C., & Navarrete, C. D. (2014). Negatively-biased credulity and the cultural evolution of beliefs. *PloS One, 9*(4). https://doi.org/10.1371/journal.pone.0095167

Funke, D. (2018, April 27). 9 ways you can help fact-checkers during a crisis. *Poynter.* https://www.poynter.org/fact-checking/2018/9-ways-you-can-help-fact-checkers-during-a-crisis/

Ghenai, A., & Mejova, Y. (2018, November 1). Fake Cures. *Proceedings of the ACM on Human-Computer Interaction.* https://dl.acm.org.remotexs.ntu.edu.sg/doi/abs/10.1145/3274327

Gneezy, U., & Imas, A. (2014). Materazzi effect and the strategic use of anger in competitive interactions. *Proceedings of the National Academy of Sciences, 111*(4), 1,334–1,337. https://doi.org/10.1073/pnas.1313789111

Gov.sg. (2020, January 23). *What you can do to protect yourself from the 2019 novel coronavirus.* https://www.gov.sg/article/what-can-you-do-to-protect-yourself-from-2019-ncov

Ho, S. S., Peh, X., & Soh, V. W. L. (2013). The cognitive mediation model: Factors influencing public knowledge of the H1N1 pandemic and intention to take precautionary behaviors. *Journal of Health Communication, 18*(7), 773–794. https://doi.org/10.1080/10810730.2012.743624

Kelly, J. R., Iannone, N. E., & McCarty, M. K. (2016). Emotional contagion of anger is automatic: An evolutionary explanation. *British Journal of Social Psychology, 55*(1), 182–191. https://doi.org/10.1111/bjso.12134

Kiely, E., & Robertson, L. (2016, November 18). *How to Spot Fake News.* FactCheck.Org. https://www.factcheck.org/2016/11/how-to-spot-fake-news/

Kok, X. (2020, January 29). "Made in China": How Wuhan coronavirus spread anti-Chinese racism like a disease through Asia. *South China Morning Post.* https://www.scmp.com/week-asia/health-environment/article/3048104/made-china-how-wuhan-coronavirus-spread-anti-chinese

Kwang, K. (2019, May 2). Facebook expands fact-checking initiative to Singapore amid challenges in other markets. *Channel NewsAsia.* https://www.channelnewsasia.com/news/singapore/facebook-fact-checking-singapore-amid-challenges-other-markets-11496900

Lewandowsky, S., Ecker, U. K. H., Seifert, C. M., Schwarz, N., & Cook, J. (2012). Misinformation and its correction: Continued influence and successful debiasing. *Psychological Science in the Public Interest, 13*(3), 106–131. https://doi.org/10.1177/1529100612451018

Lim, S. S. (2020, January 30). Commentary: Wuhan virus—when social media and chat groups complicate crisis communication. *Channel NewsAsoa.* https://www.channelnewsasia.com/news/commentary/wuhan-virus-social-media-communications-facebook-whatsapp-12364658

Lufkin, B. (2020, March 5). Coronavirus: The psychology of panic buying. *BBC News.* https://www.bbc.com/worklife/article/20200304-coronavirus-covid-19-update-why-people-are-stockpiling

Lundgren, R. E., & McMakin, A. H. (2013). Constraints to effective risk communication. In *Risk communication: A handbook for communicating environmental, safety, and health risks.* John Wiley & Sons.

MHA to look into "racist, xenophobic" remarks by religious teacher over coronavirus: Shanmugam. (2020, February 7). *Channel NewsAsia.* https://www.channelnewsasia.com/news/singapore/mha-wuhan-virus-shanmugam-abdul-halim-racist-remarks-12403812

Misleading information about smoking/vaping links to COVID-19. (2020, April 27). *Global Center for Good Governance in Tobacco Control.* https://ggtc.world/2020/04/27/misleading-information-about-smoking-vaping-links-to-covid-19/

Newman, N., Fletcher, R., Kalogeropoulos, A., & Nielsen, R. K. (2019). *Reuters Institute Digital News Report 2019.* Reuters Institute.

Oyeyemi, S. O., Gabarron, E., & Wynn, R. (2014). Ebola, Twitter, and misinformation: A dangerous combination? *The British Medical Journal, 349.* https://doi.org/10.1136/bmj.g6178

Sehlmeyer, C., Schöning, S., Zwitserlood, P., Pfleiderer, B., Kircher, T., Arolt, V., & Konrad, C. (2009). Human fear conditioning and extinction in neuroimaging: A systematic review. *PLoS ONE, 4*(6). https://doi.org/10.1371/journal.pone.0005865

Silverman, C. (2019, July 23). What to do if the older people in your life are sharing false or extreme content. *BuzzFeed News.* https://www.buzzfeednews.com/article/craigsilverman/young-people-worry-about-older-people-sharing-fake-news

SPH Magazines complies with Pofma correction order on false HardwareZone post related to the Wuhan virus. (2020, January 27). *The Straits Times.* https://www.straitstimes.com/singapore/sph-magazines-complies-with-pofma-correction-order-on-false-hardwarezone-post

Tan, H. H., Neo, L. S., & Chen, X. K. (2019, July). *Understanding why people do not intervene in the spread of fake news* [Poster]. 4th Asian Conference of Criminal & Operations Psychology, Singapore.

Tandoc, E. C., Jr. (2017, May 27). It's up to you, yes you, to stop fake news. *The Straits Times.* http://www.straitstimes.com/opinion/its-up-to-you-yes-you-to-stop-fake-news

Tandoc, E. C., Jr., Ling, R., Westlund, O., Duffy, A., Goh, D., & Zheng Wei, L. (2018). Audiences' acts of authentication in the age of fake news: A conceptual framework. *New Media & Society, 20*(8), 2,745–2,763. https://doi.org/10.1177/1461444817731756

Tay, J., Ng, Y. F., Cutter, J., & James, L. (2010). Influenza A (H1N1-2009) pandemic in Singapore—Public health control measures implemented and lessons learnt. *Annals, Academy of Medicine Singapore, 39*(4), 313-12. https://pubmed.ncbi.nlm.nih.gov/20473458/

Taylor, J. (2020, February 6). Viral hysteria: Hong Kong coronavirus panic sparks run on toilet paper. *Hong Kong Free Press HKFP*. https://www.hongkongfp.com/2020/02/06/viral-hysteria-hong-kong-coronavirus-panic-sparks-run-toilet-paper/

Thomas, Z. (2020, February 13). WHO says fake coronavirus claims causing "infodemic". *BBC News*. https://www.bbc.com/news/technology-51497800

Verduyn, P., Delvaux, E., Van Coillie, H., Tuerlinckx, F., & Van Mechelen, I. (2009). Predicting the duration of emotional experience: Two experience sampling studies. *Emotion, 9*(1), 83–91. https://doi.org/ 10.1037/a0014610

Vijaykumar, S., Nowak, G., Himelboim, I., & Jin, Y. (2018). Managing social media rumors and misinformation during outbreaks. *American Journal of Infection Control, 46*(7), 850. https://doi.org/10.1016/j.ajic.2018.03.014

Voss, C., & Raz, T. (2016). *Never split the difference: Negotiating as if your life depended on it*. Random House.

Wineburg, S., & McGrew, S. (2017). Lateral reading: Reading less and learning more when evaluating digital information. *Stanford History Education Group Working Paper No. 2017-A1*. https://dx.doi.org/10.2139/ssrn.3048994

Yoo, W., Choi, D-H., & Park, K. (2016). The effects of SNS communication: How expressing and receiving information predict MERS-preventive behavioral intentions in South Korea. *Computers in Human Behavior, 62*, 34–43. https://doi.org/10.1016/j.chb.2016.03.058

Chapter 11

# Maintaining Cyber Well-Being During a Pandemic

Jessie Janny Thenarianto

## Introduction

As the coronavirus disease 2019 (COVID-19) pandemic developed worldwide in 2020, various countries imposed physical distancing measures and lockdowns in an effort to curb the spread of the virus. As a result, a lot of activities that were normally conducted in-person (e.g., working, meeting others, learning) moved online, generating a heavy dependency on the internet and digital infrastructure. Network operators around the world, such as in the United Kingdom, Japan, and Korea, reportedly experienced up to 60% increase in internet traffic compared to before the pandemic (Organisation for Economic Co-operation and Development, 2020).

The sudden and massive adoption of the cyberspace is not without its challenges. Companies and their employees struggled to run their operations remotely through online communication channels, while students at all educational levels had to adjust the way they attended classes. Meanwhile, the increased use of computing devices and the internet took a toll on individuals' health. As screen time among adults and children surged during the pandemic, screen fatigue became a concern (Hinde, 2020). Eye strains, headaches, and overall fatigue were effects of prolonged screen use (Helander et al., 2020; Thorpe, 2020).

People were also flooded with extensive information from the online sphere. Being overloaded with COVID-19-related information during the pandemic has increased people's anxiety levels (Gao *et al.*, 2020). Misinformation surrounding the disease's prevention and treatment further created confusion, panic, and distrust in countries where the virus had spread (Blundy & Feingold, 2020).

At the same time, cybercriminals also ramped up their attacks. For example, schools, businesses, and other social groups experienced video conferencing hijacking, also more popularly known as "Zoombombing" (Morris, 2020). Organisations at the frontlines of the virus response were also targeted by cyberattacks (International Criminal Police Organisation, 2020; World Health Organisation [WHO], 2020). Such attacks have, for example, led a hospital and key COVID-19 testing site in the Czech Republic to postpone surgeries and re-route patients to another hospital (Cimpanu, 2020). Cyberattacks, particularly those targeted at essential services (e.g., hospitals, transport systems, electricity grids, telecommunication providers), could bring devastating effects on individuals and even impact the course of the pandemic (Pipikaite & Davis, 2020).

The challenges that come with cyberspace and technology use during COVID-19 highlight the need for individuals to maintain their cyber well-being. Cyber well-being or cyber wellness refers to the "positive well-being of internet users" (Ministry of Education, 2020, para. 1), and involves having an understanding of online behaviour and being able to use technology safely and responsibly (Mıhcı Türker & Kılıç Çakmak, 2019). Thus, the aim of this chapter is to provide five strategies that practitioners and policymakers as well as the general public can adopt to maintain cyber well-being during pandemics.

## Strategies to Maintain Cyber Well-Being During a Pandemic

### *Practising Good Personal Cyber Hygiene*

Individual end-users have long been considered as the weakest link in cybersecurity (CSO, 2019). Certain cyber behaviours often make individuals as well as their organisations vulnerable to attacks. Thus, an important line of defence against cyberthreats is replacing these risky behaviours with good ones (i.e., practising cyber hygiene) that help people use technology and navigate cyberspace safely.

Cyber hygiene constitutes behaviours that online users should undertake to ensure the safety of their information on their internet-enabled devices (Vishwanath *et al.*, 2020). There are a number of good cyber hygiene habits that individuals should strive to practise. First is to use strong and unique passwords. According to Yıldırım and Mackie (2019), people tend to choose and reuse weak and predictable passwords, which can be easily hacked by cybercriminals. This is because the process of thinking of a unique password and remembering it results in a large cognitive burden, which people naturally try to avoid (Blau *et al.*, 2017). One of the ways that people can use to make passwords that are hard to guess is the Schneier scheme.[1] This approach requires people to create their personal sentence and modify it into a password (Schneier, 2014). Adopting password managers to store passwords can also help ease memory burden. Second is to have up-to-date antivirus protection. To guard against computer viruses, there is a need to have robust antivirus software, keep the programme up-to-date, and run a virus scan on every external storage device that is plugged into the computing device (Vishwanath *et al.*, 2020). Third is to perform regular software updates. Software development companies often release security patches to address security vulnerabilities. Thus, it is recommended for individuals to update their software whenever patches are released.

Security practitioners and organisations also have a role to play in encouraging good cyber hygiene. This is because people tend to underestimate the probability of negative events (e.g., being a victim of a cyberattack), also known as the optimism bias, and thus overlook the importance of cyber hygiene habits (Pfleeger & Caputo, 2012). Advisories should be regularly made to encourage desirable cyber behaviour. As an example, to encourage individuals to perform software updates, we can provide clear communication on what the security patch addresses, the changes that will happen to the features, and the length of the update. This would help build users' awareness towards the importance of updating the software, and subsequently drive the "right" behaviour.

In addition, insights from the nudge theory suggest that designating a choice (e.g., a certain security measure) as the default option helps shape

---

[1]An example of the Schneier scheme usage is: "This little piggy went to market" might become "tlpWENT2m".

behaviour (Thaler & Sunstein, 2008). For instance, using multi-factor authentication (MFA) in addition to passwords helps strengthen the security of an account, yet users often perceive it as a hassle, decreasing their likelihood of using it (Blau *et al.*, 2017). Therefore, instead of letting the individual choose to opt-in to MFA, setting MFA as the default option and providing the opportunity to opt-out will increase the likelihood of individuals using it. Similarly, this strategy can also be applied to other security measures, such as making automatic software updating as the default option.

## Being Vigilant of Online Fraud Heightened by the Pandemic

Besides having good cyber hygiene habits, it is also important to be vigilant of online fraud associated with the pandemic, such as scams (e.g., e-commerce, fraudulent donation, impersonation, investment scams) and phishing attacks. In Singapore, the police handled 394 reports of scams and phishing attacks related to COVID-19 from January to April 2020 (Ministry of Home Affairs, 2020). In Australia, the Australian Competition and Consumer Commission's Scamwatch service received over 1,100 COVID-19-related scam reports from March to April 2020 (Australian Cyber Security Centre, 2020).

The upsurge of online fraud observed during the COVID-19 pandemic is not a surprise, considering that high-profile events (e.g., 2018 World Cup) and crises (e.g., 2019–2020 Australian bushfire crisis, 2008 financial crisis) in the past have often been exploited by cybercriminals. Cybercriminals take advantage of people's increased interest and concern, tricking them into their deceptive schemes (Cyber Security Agency of Singapore, 2019).

The rise in malicious cyber activities during COVID-19 can be mostly attributed to the fear of being infected, which drives people to expend great efforts to protect themselves (Taylor, 2019). For instance, fears about COVID-19, when accompanied by the shortage of masks and hand sanitisers, drove individuals to rush and buy products online, overlooking red flags of fraud. Phishing attackers preyed on people's confusion and fear, and impersonated authorities (e.g., WHO, Centers for Disease Control [CDC]) in emails to harvest personal information (Holmes, 2020). Apart from fear, other cybercriminals took advantage of people's altruism by tricking them into giving money to fraudulent donation requests.

The plethora of online fraud and people's increased vulnerability during the COVID-19 pandemic underlines the need to be vigilant when surfing and communicating online. People are encouraged to always stop and think whether something is genuine before agreeing to a request. Fraudsters commonly create a sense of urgency to rush people into making a decision and use other persuasion tactics, such as acting as a figure of authority or using cues that are familiar (Chang, 2008). To prevent phishing, for example, before clicking anything or responding to an email, people should build the habit of looking up the said organisation's website for any mention of what the email sender suggests, and even directly calling the organisation's number to verify the authenticity of the information. To prevent scams, people should keep in mind the principle of "if something seems too good to be true, it probably is" (Sammons & Cross, 2016, p. 110). When dealing with any offers online, people should investigate any claims, and be willing to challenge or reject the offer if it seems suspicious.

At the group and national levels, practitioners, organisations, and law enforcement agencies also have a part to play to prevent individuals from falling victim to online fraud. Organisational policies that help prevent fraud (e.g., disallowing sharing of links through email and providing staff with alternative platforms) need to be developed. Timely updates on the latest schemes that fraudsters have been using are also useful. For example, several countries have dedicated websites that provide updates on current fraud trends. These include Scamwatch (Australia; Australian Competition and Consumer Commission, n.d.), ScamAlert (Singapore; National Crime Prevention Council, n.d.), and Action Fraud (the United Kingdom; Action Fraud, n.d.). However, more work needs to be done to draw people's attention to these credible websites. In addition, community-wide educational campaigns on online fraud are needed to better equip the public during pandemics as well as other high-profile events and crises. For instance, the United Kingdom has the Take Five national campaign, with a simple but memorable tagline (i.e., stop-challenge-protect), which urges people to stop and think when receiving a request online (UK Finance, n.d.).

## *Following Netiquette in Online Communication*

Having good netiquette, which is the rule of online courtesy (i.e., behaviours that are acceptable when interacting with others online), is another part of cyber well-being (Mıhcı Türker & Kılıç Çakmak, 2019).

Netiquette is important to maintain a positive online environment for everyone, and even more important during a pandemic when there is a heavy reliance on online channels. This is because during a pandemic, people tend to experience high levels of psychological stress (Vinkers *et al.*, 2020), and may be easily triggered by insensitive posts online, not only further worsening their well-being, but also resulting in social tensions within the community.

Social tensions have harmful effects on the community. Increased social tensions may threaten social cohesion, which is an important ingredient for community resilience (i.e., the capacity of communities to recover from crises; Maguire & Hagan, 2007). Not only that, prior events (e.g., 2019 Hong Kong protests, 1998–2001 Poso riots, 1832 Cholera outbreak in France) have shown that tensions and mistrust between groups can lead to civil violence. In a context of a pandemic in the age of computer-mediated communication, being a good digital citizen can have far-reaching effects—it can determine the community's ability to effectively respond to the pandemic and prevent social unrest.

The general principle of netiquette is to respect others (Kayany, 2004), which includes being sensitive to the feelings of others when posting on social media. During the COVID-19 pandemic, a number of public figures and non-public figures have received backlash for making posts that are insensitive towards others. This includes saying that COVID-19 deaths are unavoidable, likening quarantine to "being in jail", and suggesting that a certain group of the population was "not making an effort to recover" (Cummins, 2020; O'Kane, 2020; Sholihyn, 2020). Others have been criticised for sharing content that was deemed disturbing, such as licking a toilet seat as part of the "coronavirus challenge", and returning juice to supermarket shelf after drinking from it while dubbing it "how to spread Wuhan virus" (Kamil, 2020; Lam, 2020). Being sensitive to others' emotions and conditions when communicating is imperative, especially in times of crisis. Sensitivity can be demonstrated by being considerate of others, showing compassion, and sharing positive content online.

At a community level, efforts to educate the public on netiquette should be done before a pandemic. This can be done by incorporating netiquette into education systems and public awareness campaigns. Singapore has included netiquette in the cyber wellness education programme, which is compulsory for students from primary school to high school levels (Ministry of Education, 2020). In this programme, students are equipped with lessons and seminars on how to develop social and cultural sensitivity as well as to show respect online (Ministry of Education, 2012). In Luxembourg, a set of netiquette principles for users navigating the country's media landscape has been developed. Users are encouraged to bear in mind that respectful coexistence in cyberspace is important and that laws also apply on social media, discouraging racist and other inappropriate content (Luxembourgish Safer Internet Centre & Press Council, 2017).

## *Minimising Screen Fatigue*

Another challenge that stems from the increased use of technology and cyberspace during a pandemic is screen fatigue. The symptoms include eye strains, mental exhaustion, and body aches (Jiang, 2020; Thorpe, 2020).

Video conferencing, in particular, was deemed taxing by many, creating the term "video call fatigue" or "Zoom fatigue" during the COVID-19 situation. Higher self-awareness and the self-imposed pressure to perform well, triggered by seeing ourselves on the screen, may have led to the fatigue (Kaye, 2020). The difficulty of processing non-verbal cues through video calls also creates added mental load (Jiang, 2020). Other explanations include the pressure to constantly gaze at other's faces and the tendency to over-schedule video calls (Fosslien & Duffy, 2020; Kaye, 2020).

Finding balance and creating boundaries is the key to manage screen fatigue. Online and offline activities should be balanced—some people may need more time to recharge after using technology. Thus, it is recommended to evaluate online activities that one undertakes (i.e., which online activity and how much of it bring positive emotions), and minimise those which negatively affect oneself. Time limits and breaks can be set, such as creating a clearly defined time allocation, even when it is a video call to socialise with family and friends, and also incorporating screen-free breaks in daily life. In addition, people can try different methods of communicating (e.g., voice calls, emails) and practise saying "no" to invites (Fosslien & Duffy, 2020).

Since screen fatigue is also accompanied by physical symptoms, people can also work on strategies to prevent and/or alleviate them. Computer eye syndrome can be relieved by following the 20-20-20 rule (i.e., taking a 20-second break to view something 20 feet away every 20 minutes of looking at a screen), having enough lighting, and reducing screen glare (American Optometric Association, n.d.), among others. Aches and pains that often follow extended periods of staring at screens can be prevented by having good sitting posture and setting reminders to take small breaks—e.g., to stand up and have a drink or do some stretching.

## *Protect Those Who Might Be Particularly Vulnerable*

In maintaining cyber well-being during a pandemic, it is also important to protect people who might be particularly vulnerable to threats online. According to the United Nations Children's Fund (UNICEF, 2020), increased internet use that accompanied the COVID-19 pandemic put children at risk of online harms, such as online sexual exploitation, cyberbullying, and online risk-taking behaviour. Besides children, elderly people who use digital devices but have limited knowledge about cyberspace are also vulnerable to cybercrimes, such as fraud (Blanco, 2020).

Protecting those who might be vulnerable online not only helps maintain their well-being and security, but also our own. For example, risky online behaviour (e.g., accidentally downloading questionable applications) that one household member engages in may endanger the data security of other members who share the same devices or network. Parents and educators need to work together to make the online sphere a safe space for children. Parents should establish ground rules (i.e., dos and don'ts) for internet use. Children should ask permission before using computing devices, comply with the rules set by the websites they are accessing, and refrain from sharing passwords or personal information online (Ministry of Education, n.d.). Other best practices include activating parental control, accompanying children when they use the internet, and having conversations with children about their media use (Ministry of Education, n.d.).

During the COVID-19 pandemic, the American Academy of Pediatrics (AAP) recommended parents to focus on creating offline experiences and ensuring that children maintain positive media use (AAP, 2020). Rather than being fixated on a certain time limit, parents can approach their children's media use using the "Three C's" framework. The framework emphasises (1) content—whether the content is educational and appropriate, (2) context—whether parents have a healthy interaction with children around media use, and (3) the child—whether the technology and digital experiences meet the needs of each child (Guernsey, 2012). To support this, educators also have a role in providing resources on offline activities, and creating quality online content for children.

As for the elderly, there is a need to encourage them to exercise caution when using technology. This includes keeping them in the loop on the potential dangers online (e.g., current fraud trends), and educating them on how they can use technology safely (e.g., refraining from giving out personal information or bank details, being wary of offers), as well as directing them to useful channels (e.g., trustworthy information sources, entertainment options). Creating digitally proficient seniors requires the support of family members. However, research has found that adult children, whom seniors most likely turn to for help, often have neither the patience nor willingness to help seniors with technology advice (Figueiredo & Aleti, 2020). Therefore, campaigns should be introduced to encourage supportive behaviour among family members of the elderly.

## Conclusion

The COVID-19 pandemic has shown that there is an increased dependency on the internet and computing devices, which emphasises the importance of maintaining one's cyber well-being. This includes protecting oneself and others from cyber threats and screen fatigue, and fostering good social relations online. In addition, limiting exposure to stress-inducing pandemic-related information (e.g., by setting time limits for pandemic-related news) is also key to safeguarding our cyber well-being while we navigate the digital world.

## Acknowledgement

The views expressed in this chapter are the author's only and do not represent the official position or view of the Ministry of Home Affairs, Singapore.

# References

Action Fraud. (n.d.). *Action fraud.* https://www.actionfraud.police.uk/

American Academy of Pediatrics. (2020, March 17). *AAP: Finding ways to keep children occupied during these challenging times.* https://services.aap.org/en/news-room/news-releases/aap/2020/aap-finding-ways-to-keep-children-occupied-during-these-challenging-times/

American Optometric Association. (n.d.). *Computer vision syndrome.* https://www.aoa.org/patients-and-public/caring-for-your-vision/protecting-your-vision/computer-vision-syndrome

Australian Competition and Consumer Commission (n.d.). *Scamwatch.* https://www.scamwatch.gov.au/

Australian Cyber Security Centre. (2020, April 20). *Threat update COVID-19 malicious cyber activity.* https://www.cyber.gov.au/sites/default/files/2020-04/ACSC-Threat-Update-COVID-19-Malicious-Cyber-Activity-20200420.pdf

Blanco, A. G. (2020, April 7). How to protect the elderly from hackers in the age of COVID-19. *BBVA.* https://www.bbva.com/en/how-to-protect-the-elderly-from-hackers-in-the-age-of-covid-19/

Blau, A., Alhadeff, A., Stern, M., Stinson, S., & Wright, J. (2017). *Deep thought: A cybersecurity story.* https://www.ideas42.org/blog/project/human-behavior-cybersecurity/deep-thought-a-cybersecurity-story/

Blundy, R., & Feingold, S. (2020, May 29). Virus misinformation fuels panic in Asia. *The Jakarta Post.* https://www.thejakartapost.com/news/2020/05/29/virus-misinformation-fuels-panic-in-asia.html

Chang, J. J. S. (2008). An analysis of advance fee fraud on the internet. *Journal of Financial Crime, 15*(1), 71–81. https://doi.org/10.1108/13590790810841716

Cimpanu, C. (2020, March 13). Czech hospital hit by cyberattack while in the midst of a COVID-19 outbreak. *ZDNet.* https://www.zdnet.com/article/czech-hospital-hit-by-cyber-attack-while-in-the-midst-of-a-covid-19-outbreak/

CSO. (2019). *The state of enterprise security: Safeguarding your organisation.* https://images.idgesg.net/assets/2019/08/security20research20study201.pdf

Cummins, E. (2020, April 22). Celebrity quarantine posts are inflaming tensions between the haves and have-nots. *Vox.* https://www.vox.com/the-highlight/2020/4/22/21228696/celebrity-quarantine-coronavirus-influencer-instagram-ellen-degeneres-arielle-charnas-class-wealth

Cyber Security Agency of Singapore. (2019, October 8). *High-profile events.* https://www.csa.gov.sg/singcert/publications/high-profile-events

Figueiredo, B., & Aleti, T. (2020, January 29). Seniors struggle with technology, and often their kids won't help. *The Conversation.* https://theconversation.com/seniors-struggle-with-technology-and-often-their-kids-wont-help-130464

Fosslien, L., & Duffy, M. W. (2020). How to combat zoom fatigue. *Harvard Business Review*. https://hbr.org/2020/04/how-to-combat-zoom-fatigue

Gao, J., Zheng, P., Jia, Y., Chen, H., Mao, Y., Chen, S., Wang, Y., Fu, H., & Dai, J. (2020). Mental health problems and social media exposure during COVID-19 outbreak. *PLoS One, 15*(4), e0231924. https://doi.org/10.1371/journal.pone.0231924

Guernsey, L. (2012). *Screen time: How electronic media—from baby videos to educational software—affects your young child*. Basic Books

Helander, M. E., Cushman, S. A., & Monnat, S. (2020, May 26). A public health side effect of the coronavirus pandemic: screen time-related eye strain and eye fatigue. *Lerner Center for Public Health Promotion*. https://lernercenter.syr.edu/wp-content/uploads/2020/05/Helander_Cushman_Monnat.pdf

Hinde, N. (2020, March 25). Screen fatigue is real. Here's how to keep tired eyes at bay. *The Huffington Post*. https://www.huffingtonpost.co.uk/entry/screen-fatigue-working-from-home_uk_5e7a0f5fc5b62f90bc51a264

Holmes, A. (2020, March 9). Email scammers are taking advantage of coronavirus fears to impersonate health officials and trick people into giving up personal information. *Business Insider Singapore*. https://www.businessinsider.sg/coronavirus-email-scam-covid-19-phishing-false-information-who-cdc-2020-2

International Criminal Police Organization. (2020, April 4). *Cybercriminals targeting critical healthcare institutions with ransomware*. https://www.interpol.int/News-and-Events/News/2020/Cybercriminals-targeting-critical-healthcare-institutions-with-ransomware

Jiang, M. (2020, April 23). The reason Zoom calls drain your energy. *BBC*. https://www.bbc.com/worklife/article/20200421-why-zoom-video-chats-are-so-exhausting

Kamil, A. (2020, March 16). TikTok user licks toilet bowl, starts "coronavirus challenge". *TODAY*. https://www.todayonline.com/singapore/tik-tok-user-licks-toilet-bowl-starts-coronavirus-challenge

Kayany, J. M. (2004). Internet etiquette (netiquette). In H. Bidgoli (Ed.), *The internet encyclopedia* (Vol. 2, pp. 274–285). John Wiley & Sons.

Kaye, L. (2020, April 21). The psychology behind "Zoom fatigue" explained. *Edge Hill University*. https://www.edgehill.ac.uk/news/2020/04/the-psychology-behind-zoom-fatigue-explained/?utm_source=ehuacuk&utm_medium=shorturl&utm_campaign=5xj

Lam, L. (2020, April 9). Teens charged after one filmed the other drinking from bottles, returning them to supermarket shelf. *Channel News Asia*. https://www.channelnewsasia.com/news/singapore/teens-drinking-juice-supermarket-video-covid-19-coronavirus-12622530

Luxembourgish Safer Internet Centre, & Press Council. (2017). *Netiquette*. https://www.netiquette.lu/index_EN.html

Maguire, B., & Hagan, P. (2007). Disasters and communities: Understanding social resilience. *The Australian Journal of Emergency Management, 22*(2), 16–20.

Mıhcı Türker, P., & Kılıç Çakmak, E. (2019). An investigation of cyber wellness awareness: Turkey secondary school students, teachers, and parents. *Computers in the Schools, 36*(4), 293–318.

Ministry of Education. (n.d.). *Parenting tips*. https://ictconnection.moe.edu.sg/cyber-wellness/for-parents/guides-and-tips/parenting-tips

Ministry of Education. (2012). *2014 syllabus cyber wellness: Secondary*. https://www.moe.gov.sg/docs/default-source/document/education/syllabuses/character-citizenship-education/files/2014-cyber-wellness-(secondary).pdf

Ministry of Education. (2020, April 27). *Practising cyber wellness*. https://beta.moe.gov.sg/programmes/cyber-wellness/

Ministry of Home Affairs. (2020, June 4). *Written reply to parliamentary question on scam cases reported since the COVID-19 started, by Mr K Shanmugam, Minister for Home Affairs and Minister for Law*. https://www.mha.gov.sg/newsroom/in-parliament/written-replies-to-parliamentary-questions/news/written-reply-to-pq-on-scam-cases-reported-since-the-covid-19-started

Morris, D. Z. (2020, April 3). Zoom meetings keep getting hacked. Here's how to prevent "Zoom bombing" on your video chats. *Fortune*. https://fortune.com/2020/04/02/zoom-bombing-what-is-meeting-hacked-how-to-prevent-vulnerability-is-zoom-safe-video-chats/

National Crime Prevention Council. (n.d.). *Let's fight scams*. https://www.scamalert.sg/

O'Kane, C. (2020, March 18). Vanessa Hudgens apologizes for "insensitive" comments about coronavirus during Instagram live video. *CBS News*. https://www.cbsnews.com/news/vanessa-hudgens-coronavirus-instagram-live-apology-social-distancing-millennials/

Organisation for Economic Co-operation and Development. (2020, May 4). *Keeping the Internet up and running in times of crisis*. http://www.oecd.org/coronavirus/policy-responses/keeping-the-internet-up-and-running-in-times-of-crisis-4017c4c9/

Pfleeger, S. L., & Caputo, D. D. (2012). Leveraging behavioral science to mitigate cyber security risk. *Computers & Security, 31*(4), 597–611. https://doi.org/10.1016/j.cose.2011.12.010

Pipikaite, A., & Davis, N. (2020, March 17). Why cybersecurity matters more than ever during the coronavirus pandemic. *World Economic Forum*. https://www.weforum.org/agenda/2020/03/coronavirus-pandemic-cybersecurity/

Sammons, J., & Cross, M. (2016). *The basics of cyber safety: Computer and mobile device safety made easy*. Elsevier

Schneier, B. (2014, March 3). *Choosing secure passwords*. https://www.schneier.com/blog/archives/2014/03/choosing_secure_1.html

Sholihyn, I. (2020, April 23). Social worker gets slammed for airing controversial opinions on migrant workers on Facebook. *AsiaOne*. https://www.asiaone.com/digital/social-worker-gets-slammed-airing-controversial-opinions-migrant-workers-facebook

Taylor, S. (2019). *The psychology of pandemics: Preparing for the next global outbreak of infectious disease.* Cambridge Scholars Publishing.

Thaler, R. H., & Sunstein, C. (2008). *Nudge: Improving decisions about health, wealth, and happiness.* Yale University Press.

Thorpe, J. R. (2020, April 17). Why do my eyes hurt? Doctors explain how the coronavirus crisis is causing strain. *Bustle*. https://www.bustle.com/p/why-do-my-eyes-hurt-doctors-explain-how-the-coronavirus-crisis-is-causing-strain-22807230

UK Finance. (n.d.). *About Take Five*. https://takefive-stopfraud.org.uk/about/take-five/

United National Children's Fund. (2020). *COVID-19 and its implications for protecting children online.* https://www.unicef.org/documents/covid-19-and-implications-protecting-children-online

Vinkers, C. H., van Amelsvoort, T., Bisson, J. I., Branchi, I., Cryan, J. F., Domschke, K., Howes, O. D., Manchia, M., Pinto, L., de Quervain, D. Schmidt, M. V., & van der Wee, N. (2020). Stress resilience during the coronavirus pandemic. *European Neuropsychopharmacology, 35*, 12–16. https://doi.org/10.1016/j.euroneuro.2020.05.003

Vishwanath, A., Neo, L. S., Goh, P., Lee, S., Khader, M., Ong, G., & Chin, J. (2020). Cyber hygiene: The concept, its measure, and its initial tests. *Decision Support Systems, 128*, 113160. https://doi.org/10.1016/j.dss.2019.113160

World Health Organisation. (2020, April 23). *WHO reports fivefold increase in cyberattacks, urges vigilance* [Press release]. https://www.who.int/news-room/detail/23-04-2020-who-reports-fivefold-increase-in-cyber-attacks-urges-vigilance

Yıldırım, M., & Mackie, I. (2019). Encouraging users to improve password security and memorability. *International Journal of Information Security, 18*(6), 741–759.

# Chapter 12

# Crisis Management and Communication During a Pandemic: Some Thoughts

Damien D. Cheong and Stephanie Neubronner

## Introduction

At the time of writing, the COVID-19 pandemic that has engulfed the world since early 2020 shows no signs of abating. Medical experts predict that this pandemic will not be diminished in the short-term (Chong, 2020). The fallout from the pandemic is obvious. In addition to causing a massive strain on the public health resources of many countries, employment, businesses, travel, trade, and even human interactions have been adversely affected.

Dealing with a crisis of this nature and magnitude is expectedly challenging. This is because various nodes and sectors within a state are all interconnected in a complex system, and the state is also connected to the world, which further increases the overall complexities. So how should states deal with this multi-faceted crisis, and how should they handle crisis communications given that communication has become vital to overall crisis management? This chapter argues that states must firstly treat a pandemic like a national security challenge, as doing so will shape both crisis management and communication strategies.

## Treating a Pandemic as a National Security Challenge

Many states often treat a pandemic as a public health issue. This could be due to many factors, including the availability of resources, governance structures, and other domestic constraints (Davies, n.d.). However, a pandemic has the potential to decimate not just a state's public health sector, but its economic and social sectors as well. Furthermore, a state's engagement with other states could also be affected. Such wide-reaching implications suggest that pandemics must be treated as a national security challenge (Monaco, 2020). Treating a pandemic as a national security challenge will invariably determine how a state manages the crisis, including its communication approaches.

## Crisis Management must be Flexible, Coordinated and Involve all Sectors

Singapore's experience with the Severe Acute Respiratory Syndrome (SARS) epidemic resulted in the development of approaches that have enabled it to deal with Novel Influenza A (H1N1), Middle East Respiratory Syndrome (MERS), and now Coronavirus Disease 2019 (COVID-19) (Kurohi, 2020). The key principles and points have been extracted and reproduced here from three documents: (1) the 2007 Monetary Authority of Singapore (MAS) Report on *Preparedness for Avian Influenza Pandemic* (Monetary Authority of Singapore, 2007), (2) the 2009 Ministry of Home Affairs (MHA) Report on *Preparing for a Human Influenza Pandemic in Singapore* (Ministry of Home Affairs, 2009), and (3) the 2014 Ministry of Health (MOH) Report on *Pandemic Readiness And Response Plan for Influenza and Other Acute Respiratory Diseases* (Ministry of Health, 2014).

It is highly recommended that readers access the full (publicly available) documents for an elaboration of the points. It should be noted that Singapore's approach is tailored to its circumstances and context, and should not be perceived as replicable in every state.[1]

### *Nature of the Pandemic*

The basic assumption about pandemics is their unpredictability. Severity would be highly dependent on "the speed and ease of human-to-human

---

[1] The United States, for example, has also published its response plans/approaches on the Centers for Disease Control and Prevention website (Centers for Disease Control and Prevention, 2017).

transmission of the virus and its lethality" (MHA, 2009, p. 7). The MOH and MHA reports caution that information about a new pandemic will be scarce (MHA, 2009; MOH, 2014), and as such, "it will take some time to determine both its speed of transmission and lethality" (MHA, 2009, p. 20).

Furthermore, it should be assumed that "economic and social life" will be adversely affected (MHA, 2009, p. 7). Specifically, states could experience:

> A sharp fall-off in domestic demand as consumers refrain from leaving home due to fear of infection and consequently reduce spending; supply-side effects arising from reduced productivity and disruptions to cross-border regional production networks; and external demand effects due to a synchronised slowdown in global demand and possible spillover effects from increased volatility in financial markets. (MAS, 2007, p. 2)

Local business operations will also suffer disruptions as individuals fall sick or die (especially staff), or refrain from participating in regular (outdoor) activities (MAS, 2007).

## *Guiding Principle*

Based on the nature of the pandemic, crisis mitigation efforts must be focused on minimising impact and accelerating recovery (MHA, 2009). To achieve this, the approach requires "coordinated national preparations, a flexible plan to guide decisive response and continued collaboration among entities within and beyond Singapore" (MHA, 2009, p. 7).

## *Approach*

Six key approaches are identified to actualise the abovementioned approach (MHA, 2009, pp. 7–8):

1. "Whole-of-Singapore" approach.
2. Close collaboration between the government and the private sector.
3. An informed and prepared public.
4. Rapid and decisive government actions.
5. Collaboration with the international community.
6. Flexibility in national response.

As the pandemic, like any crisis, would go through stages, it is prudent to develop plans at each stage (MHA, 2009, p. 9; MOH, 2014, pp. 4–5, 7–11):

a) Pre-pandemic stage: To strengthen national preparedness by developing plans for health and non-health issues that will surface during a pandemic.
b) Pandemic outside Singapore: To delay the import of pandemic influenza that occurs in other countries.
c) Initial stage of pandemic in Singapore: To take tough measures to slow the spread of the virus once initial cases are identified in the community.
d) Widespread pandemic in Singapore: To mitigate human suffering as well as the impact on social structures and the economy; to sustain the population by maintaining core government operations and essential services provided by the private sector.

## Crisis Communications Need to be Prompt, Well Informed and Balanced

Communication is, expectedly, critical at every stage of the crisis. For the purposes of this chapter, we focus on stages (b), (c), and (d). Beyond communicating about responses, an important aspect of communication is to focus on maintaining social cohesion and unity during the crisis. To ensure appropriate public action, crisis communications need to be disseminated in a timely manner, while ensuring the clarity and decisiveness of the message is not lost. Doing so will help minimise the risk of rumour mongering, preserve trust in the government, and also maintain social order.

### *Providing Frequent and Transparent Updates*

The frequent virtual press conferences held by Singapore's multi-ministry task force set up to direct the government's response to the COVID-19 pandemic has allowed for detailed explanations and announcements to be communicated to Singaporeans in a direct and effective manner.

The daily updates published on the Singapore government's dedicated website on the COVID-19 situation that details the various announcements, press releases, and other government updates about the unfolding situation further helped communicate essential information to the Singaporean populace in a quick and straightforward way. By releasing details such as updates on cases and known clusters, as well as being forthcoming about issues such as the situation in foreign worker dormitories has shown how the Singapore government has been managing the evolving situation in a transparent manner.

## *Ensuring Consistency and Credibility*

Having information released by various ministries all accessible on the same webpage dedicated to the COVID-19 situation in Singapore, which also had links to other useful resources individuals might require assistance with or have questions about (e.g., how to help seniors go digital, or details about what the circuit breaker measures mean), ensured information was not only made publicly available, but was also easy to access and digest.

Additionally, indicating links to the Factually website[2] on the government's one-stop website on the COVID-19 situation, where clarifications on misinformation and corrections regarding falsehoods that had been spreading could be found, helped reinforce the need to prevent the spread of misinformation.

Maintaining the consistency of messages, coupled with the use of infographics and explainers that were available on the government's COVID-19 website, further highlighted the whole-of-government approach that was being implemented to combat the pandemic. Such clear and consistent communication not only preserved Singaporeans' trust in the government, but also made it easier for Singaporeans to understand and make necessary adjustments. The benefits of such a communication

---

[2]According to former Communications and Information Minister Yaacob Ibrahim, the state-run Factually website has been in operation since 2012 and is aimed at clarifying "widespread or common misperceptions of government policy, or incorrect assertions on matters of public concern that can harm Singapore's social fabric". Responding to Non-Constituency MP Leon Perera, who wanted to know how the webpage selected falsehoods to respond to in Parliament in March 2017, Dr. Yaccob said that "this [was] part of the Government's efforts to ensure Singaporeans have access to accurate information on important matters" (Lee, 2017).

strategy were evident when the Singapore government implemented strict measures on a large scale and at very short notice, executing the Circuit Breaker in an efficient and effective manner.

## Utilising Various Communication Channels

The use of multiple channels and platforms to disseminate crisis communications has helped Singapore's response to the COVID-19 pandemic. By using WhatsApp to disseminate information, as well as tapping on social media (e.g., Facebook), and getting the media to help disseminate succinct and accurate information, the reach of such communications was not only enhanced, but was made more comprehensible, ensuring different segments of the population received the messages in a manner they understood.

Such agile methods of communicating not only indicates the Singapore government's ability to adjust to meet current needs, but also ensures that the rationales behind decisions made were clear and transparent. Publishing frequent updates through the various channels further provided the Singapore government with platforms that could be used to address the public's concerns and assure its citizens that plans were in place to safeguard their well-being.

## Addressing Citizens' Concerns

Immediately after the Ministry of Health (MOH) raised Singapore's Disease Outbreak Response System Condition (DORSCON) risk assessment level from "Yellow" to "Orange" in February 2020, crazed panic buying of essentials such as rice and toilet paper occurred. It was the prompt, accurate, direct and balanced messages published by the Singapore government that helped restore order, allaying citizen's concerns that there would be shortages of essential items.

The four additional Budgets[3] that amount close to $100 billion, or 20% of Singapore's GDP ("Fortitude Budget to support Singaporeans", 2020b),

---

[3] The $6.4 billion Unity Budget was announced on 18 February. The supplementary $48.4 billion Resilience Budget was announced on 26 March 2020 and the $5.1 billion Solidarity Budget was announced on 6 April to enhance the measures previously announced (Zhou, 2020). On 26 May 2020, a fourth support package in the form of the $33 billion Fortitude Budget was announced ("Fortitude Budget to support Singaporeans", 2020b).

which were announced to "care for and support all Singaporeans at every stage of their lives" and "stabilise, grow and transform the economy so that Singaporeans can stay employed, and have access to better opportunities" also helped alleviate fears Singaporeans had resulting from the disruptions caused by the pandemic (Government of Singapore, 2020b; Zhou, 2020). Such initiatives and aid packages helped impart the message that the government had things under control and was aware of the concerns its citizens had. And, by announcing such measures in a timely and clear manner, with the aid of social media and different platforms to disseminate the relevant information, trust and transparency, which are critical in times of crisis, could be reinforced.

### *The Importance of Balanced Messages*

The World Health Organisation (WHO) has praised Singapore for its initial response to the pandemic ("WHO impressed by Singapore", 2020). Policy observers have further attributed Singapore's success to the combination of three critical factors: (1) strong economic policy, (2) assured political leadership, and (3) evidence-based knowledge.

Still, in the age of social media, credibility is not guaranteed and is based entirely on what makes sense to individual consumers. The content being disseminated thus needs to be packaged appropriately and effectively to ensure the right kind of engagement and responses are elicited. Being prompt and accurate with updates and directives also needs to be accompanied by balanced messages.

Ensuring crisis communications are relatable, authentic, and appropriately address concerns is key. Without which, it will be hard to convince the public to get on board and follow measures that have been implemented. People look to their leaders to see if they can understand their struggles. Thus, having empathy, being open and having regular communication all the while ensuring accountability will help leaders communicate messages that are sensible and well balanced.

Amid the chaos brought about by the COVID-19 pandemic, German Chancellor Angela Merkel and New Zealand Prime Minister Jacinda Ardern have shined in appealing to their people based on their unique leadership styles. Merkel's calm, rational assurances, as well as her goal-oriented and emotional approach were crucial at a time of rising panic, and has helped Germany deal with the outbreak better than many other countries.

Likewise, Ardern's clear, consistent, and empathetic style has resonated with New Zealanders on an emotional level, deepening the high level of trust and confidence New Zealanders have in her. Ardern's ability to adapt and embrace new media, using Facebook Live Chat to connect with New Zealanders on a more personal level, on top of her daily formal briefings, has also helped her address concerns and communicate with New Zealanders in a relatable and yet factual manner.

## Crisis Communication should not Omit Community Centric Messages

When dealing with crises, it is easy to focus on more obvious and pressing aspects such as the operationalisation of government directives. However, the maintenance of societal cohesion should not be forgotten.

### *Emphasising Unity and Social Harmony*

To keep societies together, especially in times of crisis, it is essential that crisis communications emphasise the importance of unity and social harmony. Messages should also include ways individuals can tackle the crisis at a personal level, thus acknowledging not only the physical, but mental toll such crisis situations pose.

Humanising the crisis situation, giving practical examples of how to maintain social contact and togetherness, despite observing social distancing, because sharing and keeping in touch are precisely what is needed in times of immense stress and uncertainty, needs to be included in crisis communications to achieve a holistic approach to tacking pandemics.

Examples of how positive community-centric messages can be spread during a crisis include initiatives such as Clap For #SGUnited, a campaign inspired by the United Kingdom's moving #ClapforNHS, which has caught on in Madrid, Amsterdam, and New York, where millions stood at their front doors and balconies to cheer on frontline workers ("Clap for #SGUnited", 2020), and Sing Together Singapore, the "massive 'karaoke' session" that rallied Singaporeans together to show their "support and appreciation for … healthcare and migrant workers", and also "encourage all Singaporeans to keep their spirits high and to stay united as everyone remain[ed] at home during the extended circuit breaker period" ("Join the entire nation in", 2020a).

Using social media to publicise such events, creating hashtags,[4] and having the government, Singaporean ministers, local celebrities, and the media industry support such events emphasises how despite being physically apart, it was still possible to come together and participate in the sing-along to show support for those on the frontline, as well as migrant workers who have been hardest hit by the coronavirus in Singapore. When videos of people clapping, cheering, and singing at their balconies were captured and shared on social media for both Clap For #SGUnited and Sing Together Singapore, individuals interviewed by *The Straits Times* said that the response was "amazing", "encouraging", and "heartening", emphasising the strength of community spirit in Singapore (Ho, 2020).

Such easy ways of fostering connections and the positivity such messages carry, need to be emphasised to ensure the community sticks together and keeps their morale up, while safeguarding its emotional support networks. Such scenes were, however, in sharp contrast with what occurred in the United States. President Trump's reference to the coronavirus as the "China Virus" was arguably a contributory factor in the stigmatisation of individuals of Asian descent, particularly Asian Americans (Yam, 2020). In less than half a month since the *Stop Asian American and Pacific Islander (AAPI) Hate* website was launched, more than 1,000 Asian Americans[5] had logged on to its website to report stories of being verbally and physically attacked (De Souza, 2020). Reports of Asian Americans being shunned, spat at, and being targets of racist sentiments were also prevalent, resulting in the spread of fear and panic within the Asian community (Aratani, 2020; Lee, 2020).

By fostering social cohesion, communities can stand up to the anxiety, division, isolation, and prejudice crises bring along with them. Genuine connections also build a stronger and more resilient society that is able to overcome the darkest and most difficult challenges posed by crises, which impact far beyond the human tragedy of lives lost.

---

[4]For the biggest singalong event ever hosted in Singapore, Sing Together Singapore, the hashtags #singtogetherSG, #SingaporeTogether and #stayhomeforSG were created and the public was encouraged to take to their balconies and windows to sing the popular NDP song, Home and upload clips of their performances.

[5]Figure is as of 30 March 2020. The website was created on 19 March and thus, translates to about 100 reports a day since the website's inception.

## What Government Leaders Can Do

Leaders such as Singapore's Prime Minister Lee Hsien Loong (PM Lee) have made it a point to be frank and communicate openly and directly to the Singaporean populace, explaining the situation and also what might lie ahead. PM Lee also gave practical advice as to how to "take sensible precautions, help one another, stay calm, and carry on with … lives", going forward (Government of Singapore, 2020a). In an address made on 8 February 2020, PM Lee reiterated that Singaporeans had to do their part:

> One, observe personal hygiene—wash your hands often, and avoid touching your eyes or face unnecessarily. Two, take your temperature twice daily. And three, if you are not well, please avoid crowded places and see a doctor immediately. These simple steps do not take much effort, but if we all do them, they will go a long way towards containing the spread of the virus. (Government of Singapore, 2020a)

Providing simple and helpful information as to how to take action, while stressing the significance of social cohesion and psychological resilience, and indicating how to "take courage and see through this stressful time together" are relatable and easy to understand. Cautionary advice against behaviours that could incite even more fear or panic in the community, such as hoarding face masks or food and spreading rumours online, provides another way of ensuring crisis communication also helps push out community-centric messages (Government of Singapore, 2020a). Giving examples of individuals who have stepped forward to contribute to the nation's psychological resilience and the social compact is another way of encouraging individuals to step up, and remain united and resolute in times of crisis.

# Conclusion

The COVID-19 pandemic will be with us for the foreseeable future. And, as the risk of new pandemics is likely (Yeung, 2019), it is perhaps timely to think about how crisis management and communication strategies can be improved *vis-à-vis* pandemics.

By treating pandemics as a national security challenge, multi-faceted crises, such as those presented by COVID-19, can then be handled in a manner that ensures a state's civil, economic, social and psychological defence. An effective and well-balanced crisis management and communications strategy that addresses the interconnectedness of states internally as well as externally needs to be formulated and, when necessary, executed in an efficient manner. Doing so will better prepare states for the disruptions caused by pandemics, reducing the strains placed on public health resources, employment, businesses, travel, trade, and even human interactions.

# References

Aratani, L. (2020, March 24). Coughing while Asian: Living in fear as racism feeds off coronavirus panic. *The Guardian.* https://www.theguardian.com/world/2020/mar/24/coronavirus-us-asian-americans-racism

Centers for Disease Control and Prevention. (2017, June 15). *National Pandemic Strategy.* https://www.cdc.gov/flu/pandemic-resources/national-strategy/index.html

Chong, C. (2020, June 1). Unlike SARS, COVID-19 will be here for some time: Experts. *The Straits Times.* https://www.straitstimes.com/singapore/unlike-sars-covid-19-will-be-here-for-some-time-experts

Clap for #SGUnited: Cheer for our healthcare heroes from your window tonight in Singapore. (2020, March 30). *City Nomads.* https://citynomads.com/clap-for-sgunited-cheer-for-healthcare-heroes-singapore/

Davies, S. E. (n.d.). *National Security and Pandemics.* https://www.un.org/en/chronicle/article/national-security-and-pandemics

De Souza, A. (2020, April 1). Asian Americans tell harrowing stories of abuse amid coronavirus outbreak in the US. *The Straits Times.* https://www.straitstimes.com/world/united-states/asian-americans-tell-harrowing-stories-of-abuse-amid-coronavirus-outbreak-in-the

Government of Singapore. (2020a, February 10). *PM Lee: The COVID-19 situation in Singapore.* https://www.gov.sg/article/pm-lee-hsien-loong-on-the-covid-19-situation-in-singapore

Government of Singapore. (2020b, June 5). *Budget 2020: Advancing as One Singapore.* https://www.gov.sg/features/budget2020

Highlights: Heng Swee Keat delivers Fortitude Budget to support Singaporeans amid COVID-19 pandemic. (2020b, May 26). *Channel NewsAsia.* https://www.channelnewsasia.com/news/singapore/live-dpm-heng-swee-keat-fortitude-fourth-budget-covid-19-12769238

Ho, O. (2020, March 30). Singapore gives those on coronavirus front lines a round of applause. *The Straits Times.* https://www.straitstimes.com/singapore/singapore-gives-coronavirus-frontliners-a-round-of-applause

Join the entire nation in singing Home to thank healthcare, migrant workers. (2020a, April 23). *Channel NewsAsia.* https://cnalifestyle.channelnewsasia.com/trending/sing-together-singapore-home-12670262

Kurohi, R. (2020, February 2). Fighting the Wuhan virus: How Singapore tackled previous epidemics. *The Straits Times.* https://www.straitstimes.com/singapore/how-singapore-tackled-previous-epidemics

Lee, P. (2017, March 2). Factually website clarifies "widespread" falsehoods. *The Straits Times.* https://www.straitstimes.com/singapore/factually-website-clarifies-widespread-falsehoods

Lee, B. Y. (2020, February 18). How COVID-19 coronavirus is uncovering anti-Asian racism. *Forbes.* https://www.forbes.com/sites/brucelee/2020/02/18/how-covid-19-coronavirus-is-uncovering-anti-asian-racism/#4021753729a6

Ministry of Health. (2014, April). *MOH Pandemic Readiness and Response Plan for Influenza and Other Acute Respiratory Diseases.* https://www.moh.gov.sg/docs/librariesprovider5/diseases-updates/interim-pandemic-plan-public-ver-_april-2014.pdf

Ministry of Home Affairs. (2009). *Preparing for a Human Influenza Pandemic in Singapore.* https://www.mha.gov.sg/docs/default-source/others/nsfpfinalversion.pdf

Monaco, L. (2020, March 3). Pandemic disease is a threat to national security. *Foreign Affairs.* https://www.foreignaffairs.com/articles/2020-03-03/pandemic-disease-threat-national-security

Monetary Authority of Singapore. (2007, July). *Preparedness for Avian Influenza Pandemic and Security Threats.* https://www.mas.gov.sg/-/media/MAS/About-MAS/Monographs-and-information-papers/MAS-BCM-Info-Paper-2007.pdf

WHO impressed by how Singapore handles coronavirus outbreak. (2020, February 20). *The Straits Times.* https://www.straitstimes.com/singapore/who-impressed-by-how-spore-handles-outbreak

Yam, K. (2020, March 17). Trump tweets about coronavirus using term "Chinese Virus". *NBC News.* https://www.nbcnews.com/news/asian-america/trump-tweets-about-coronavirus-using-term-chinese-virus-n1161161

Yeung, J. (2019, September 18). The risk of a global pandemic is growing—and the world isn't ready, experts say. *CNN.* https://edition.cnn.com/2019/09/18/health/who-pandemic-report-intl-hnk-scli/index.html

Zhuo, T. (2020, April 7). $60b help to fight Covid-19. *The Straits Times.* https://www.straitstimes.com/singapore/60b-help-to-fight-covid-19

# Section 4

# Organisational Related Issues

# Chapter 13

# How to Enhance Organisation Functioning in a Pandemic: COVID-19 Lessons in Leadership

Paul Englert

## Introduction

*"Do not pray for an easy life, pray for the strength to endure a difficult one"*

— *Bruce Lee*

The COVID-19 pandemic has brought about an unprecedented change for organisations. With social distancing mandated in most countries (Dunford *et al.*, 2020), resulting in new working from home protocols (Ministry of Manpower, 2020), organisations have had to adapt to new ways of operating. Downsizing of organisations has occurred at a rapid rate, a rate unseen since the great depression (Iacurci, 2020). There is even talk that the economic shift will be more significant in Europe than at any other time over the past 300 years (Riley, 2020).

Future leaders will now need to demonstrate skills in making decisions about how to restructure an organisation in the face of pandemics, and do so with the compassion expected at such difficult times. These same leaders must then show a different set of skills in being able to galvanise the staff that remain, around a vision for the future.

While many organisations have policies for events as irregular as natural disasters or more regular events such as bereavement or maternity leave, pandemics were not on most company's risk radar before COVID-19 (EY Global, 2020). As such, the pandemic has exposed gaps in organisational policies and leadership practices. Employees who experienced the pandemic directly were naturally bewildered and lost, and looked for leadership to help guide them through the process. Restructured jobs have resulted in employees— who may have been with the company for their working life—moving out of the organisation; indeed, in some cases, displaced workers may represent intergenerational employees (Baron, & Francois, 2020). Employees that remain have the potential to develop survivor syndrome (Nielson, 2020), wondering why they were fortunate enough to stay employed.

The COVID-19 pandemic has, nevertheless, provided an opportunity for leaders to stress-test their capability to operate in a crisis. The lessons learnt through COVID-19 are not, however, new. Instead, what leaders experienced during the pandemic is an extreme test of their leadership capabilities. Fortunately, there is a large body of work that leaders can draw upon at this time to facilitate the development of leadership skills required to navigate the difficult economic and social times successfully.

Preparing to lead through a pandemic is, in essence, equivalent to being a great leader. A leader is not the person who can lead when times are easy. Instead, a pandemic is an example of the exact time that organisations require leadership, and it is in stressful times that the skills of leaders are most tested. Leadership is necessary for a crisis, and it is leadership that has perhaps the most critical role to play in enhancing the functioning of an organisation at the time of a pandemic (Teo *et al.*, 2017).

Leaders need more than a hotch-botch of different ideas to help them to prepare for the next crisis. In a busy world, what is required are the fundamental skills that will act like Archimedes levers, achieving an excellent outcome with a targeted focus. In the words often attributed to Winston Churchill, "We should never let a good crisis go to waste". The COVID-19 pandemic has highlighted the skills required by organisational leaders in a crisis, and it is these skills that are now necessary for leaders to cultivate and master as they prepare for what will be the inevitable next upheaval.

# Leadership Lesson 1: Authentic Leaders Demonstrate Vulnerability and Transparency

The leaders who have fared well during the COVID-19 crisis have tended to be those leaders who demonstrated a strong sense of authenticity (Koehn, 2020). News clips of leaders who expressed the emotional pain of having to make people redundant such that others would keep their jobs had a positive effect on both employees and the wider public (cf. Gallo, 2020). Society has lauded leaders who had a clear sense of both their values and how those values translate to effectively being able to negotiate social and economic change brought about by the COVID-19 pandemic (cf. McCarthy, 2020). The public wants leaders who have the integrity of character, such that their actions and words align.

Authenticity allows these leaders to demonstrate a vulnerability that is important for creating a connection with others. Vulnerability, correctly shown, has been demonstrated to have many positive outcomes for leaders (Bunker, 1997). A key finding from the research is that vulnerability builds trust between leaders and their followers (Nienaber *et al.*, 2015). In times of crisis, maximising trust between management and direct reports may well be the essential attribute that leaders can cultivate with their team (Burke *et al.*, 2007).

Vulnerability also comes in many varieties. For some, that vulnerability will include emotional reactions, such as crying. For others, the demonstration of vulnerability is through forthright and somewhat stoic speech (Ladkin & Taylor, 2010). The key, however, is that the vulnerability is authentic.

Authentic leadership will also allow leaders to show an appropriate level of transparency with staff. Survivors of the restructure, and those affected, will want clarity on what is happening and the rationale for decisions. Authentic leaders will have the capacity to front such talks, and not shy away from direct and honest communication, especially in times of crisis.

Authentic leadership is especially important to cultivate in countries where there can be a power distance gap, such as Singapore (House *et al.*, 2013). Often leaders in these countries have a mental schema as to how a leader should or should not behave (House *et al.*, 2013). The models adopted in countries with a high-power distance gap often create a distance between a leader and a follower that may make it difficult for authentic connection. Leaders ushering statements that are somewhat contrived from the way one would typically behave will lack the authenticity to lead with credibility.

At the heart of authentic leadership is having a deep understanding and appreciation of one's values and living accordingly (Gardner *et al.*, 2005). Self-knowledge is the foundation of the authentic leader (Gardner *et al.*, 2005). Leaders wanting to prepare for the next pandemic need to take the time now to deepen their understanding of who they are and what their values are. For example, questions that leaders may ask themselves might include: Given the importance I place on fairness, how would I behave should this situation arise again? What strengths do I bring to a crisis? What are my possible weak points, and can I address any gaps I have? Developing authenticity will require leaders to engage in self-reflection proactively, and have an established sense of self that is comfortable being on display during a crisis.

Authentic leadership in action will require dealing with people with transparency and honesty to a level that is not self-protective, but reflects the gravity of the situation. Authentic leaders have the character to deliver unsettling messages with compassion but without trying to water the message down. Again, as we have learnt through the COVID-19 pandemic, this level of authenticity is especially critical in a crisis.

## Leadership Lesson 2: Lead with a Focus on Creativity, Not Productivity

For many leaders, their leadership effectiveness is measured using traditional productivity metrics. These metrics include perceived tangible measures of performance, such as the time at the desk, or quantity, not the quality of output (Hughes *et al.*, 1999). Even more contemporary measures of organisational performance, such as organisational citizenship behaviours (Podsakoff *et al.*, 2009) and adaptive performance (Pulakos *et al.*, 2000) often fail to encapsulate the practices required of leaders to lead through a crisis.

A pandemic represents a time when standard solutions will not suffice. As a result, leaders need to take the time to both read and acquire new information as well as the time to process this information to formulate a vision to then lead employees through that vision. The process of bringing in novel information to come up with new solutions is at the heart of the creative process, a process that is not well respected in many organisations (Paulus, 2000). For example, the creative process will require that a leader has the time to think, and that process will often appear, to an outsider, to be time away from actually working. Thinking time will often involve solitary activities to encourage thought, such as long walks and even long baths (Reeves & Fuller, 2020). Alternatively, it may include social activities such as discussion and debate with colleagues so that novel and practical ideas are allowed to germinate; a style of work known as deep work (Newport, 2016).

Deep work is not something that many leaders are either familiar with or find comfortable. They enjoy the process of being busy. The optimal time for deep work is often seen as three to four hours a day (cf. Newport, 2017). Leaders need to cultivate time not only for their deep work and for appropriate levels of deep work in their team. Allowance for deep work will require a different approach to the management of staff as well as expectations on leaders.

Performance measurement for many jobs, especially leadership, is no longer quantitative. Instead, performance assessment is by the quality of the output (Landy & Conte, 2018). Work arrangements are flexible both in the place of work, such as at home and the time of day one chooses to work. Leading in a post-COVID-19 environment will require leaders to have the openness to embrace individual variance in working style while maintaining standards of work output. To achieve goals that are not as clearly defined as objectives of the past will require leaders who can reframe productivity within the language and metrics of creativity.

## Leadership Lesson 3: Leaders Create a Vision

As discussed, the output of creativity will be a clear vision for the organisation. The ability to have a vision is often synonymous with leadership and is recognised by researchers as one of the core components of effective leadership (Englert *et al.*, 2006; House & Shamir, 1993; Ireland & Hitt, 2005). The failure of world leaders, such as in the United States and the United Kingdom, to articulate a vision during COVID-19 was cited as a central cause of the catastrophic outcomes that resulted, and more importantly, could have been avoided (Horton, 2020; "The Coronavirus pandemic", 2020).

Many leaders have not had the opportunity to cultivate this skill set, and their leadership focus is more one of risk management rather than strategic growth (Reeves & Fuller, 2020). The failure to develop a vision will be especially the case in large organisations which have a robust hierarchal structure. In large hierarchical organisations, devolution of visioning often occurs, and all, but the most senior managers may have to implement other's vision. One can contrast hierarchical organisations with lean start-ups, which are often defined by their commitment to the vision (Lewis & Clark, 2020).

The visioning skills described do not have to result in grandiose plans. The vision can be something as simple as estimates on how a pandemic might affect an organisation or a given department, and actions to take to minimise the impact. The key is to be able to create a vision that gives staff a sense of purpose and security. Creating clarity for staff who are working through a crisis, will, by necessity, be a core function of all levels of leadership in the future.

To understand the value of the ability to create a vision for employees to follow, we can draw upon foundational leadership theories, such as path-goal leadership (House, 1971). Under path-goal leadership, the leader's role is to create the goal and a clear path for the individual's goal attainment. Employees affected by a pandemic need as much clarity and security as possible about their future state. They need to understand what the new way of working will look like, how the business will operate under this new normal and what they will need to do to get there.

To be a strategically visionary leader, leaders need to cultivate the skill of visioning in the time outside of a crisis. Questions a leader may ask themselves include: If I had to pivot this business, what would be involved? What significant trends do I foresee impacting this business, and how do I prepare for them? What is a plan for which I am happy to take ownership? Developing strategies in this way will help leaders not only to create a vision, but also have the feeling of ownership required to manifest the plan, by cultivating the people.

## Leadership Lesson 4: Aim for Operational Excellence to Ensure Organisational Success

A vision without the ability to implement on that vision is idealism (Hitt *et al.*, 2012). For this reason, operational excellence, together with a vision, is critical for the organisation success. Thus, operational excellence demonstrated by the leader may be the defining characteristic of a successful organisation (Englert *et al.*, 2006). Trying to prepare during a pandemic is akin to repairing a plane while flying, while theoretically possible it is not advisable. What is required is for one to ensure the aircraft is flightworthy before the take-off. However, unprepared is precisely the position that many companies found themselves in during COVID-19. A survey conducted mid-way through the COVID-19 outbreak found that only 38% of companies felt well prepared to cope during a pandemic ("Companies still not prepared", 2020). COVID-19 has highlighted just how unprepared many organisations are to deal with large-scale disruption, despite the rhetoric of being agile and adaptable (Worley & Jules 2020).

Leaders that have emphasised operational excellence, rather than accepting processes and procedures that are merely good enough, are likely to have transitioned well through the stages of the pandemic (Jandhyala, 2020). Organisations that were quickly able to work remotely, due to sufficient preparation with systems and processes, experienced minimal downtime through the pandemic. An unambiguous working from home policy and technology aids to assist working from home was evident in organisations well prepared for the pandemic. For other organisations, the pandemic highlighted weaknesses in their adaptability and forced rapid, and often the disorganised implementation of technological solutions that could have been in place well in advance (cf. Marr, 2020).

Systems have long been the backbone of the organisation. People do not rise to the aspirations of their goals; they fall to the quality of their systems (Clear, 2018). The importance of systems is as significant for the individual as it is for the organisation. A crisis is not the time to perfect one's operational system. An analogy from fighting is quite apt for illustrating this point. Fighters train so that on the day of the competition, their behaviour is locked-in. The day of the fight is not the time to be practising new techniques.

Systems and routine are especially important during a pandemic when working from home may be the norm. Leaders need to make sure that everyone is connecting much like they would at work, not too little and not too often. Indeed, one of the new symptoms that came from the current COVID-19 crisis is the idea of "Zoom fatigue" (Jiang, 2020). Zoom is a communication application that became popular at the time of the crisis due to its functionality for video conferencing. However, for some people, the level of interaction via Zoom was more than they could handle or desired. Systems will thus include not only the technology to adapt to a pandemic, but also the policies and procedures on the effective use of the technology to enhance organisational outcomes without overtaxing individuals.

## Leadership Lesson 5: The Need to Develop Emotional Intelligence

The concept of emotional intelligence (EI) is not accepted entirely in the scientific literature (Zeidner *et al.*, 2004). Some argue that EI is the relabelling of traits such as neuroticism and agreeableness. For these researchers, EI it is not science but the commercialisation of science (Zeidner *et al.*, 2001).

However, the practical benefit of EI for leaders is difficult to overstate. Many studies indicate that a core skill that differentiates effective leaders from those who may be less effective, is their EI. The ability to operate as an authentic leader, to create a clear vision, and to deliver that vision, will ultimately come down to their ability to work effectively with their own emotions while being mindful of other emotional states.

Three key competencies capture the essence of EI. The first is the capacity to understand and express one's own emotions (Palmer *et al.*, 2008). Understanding one's own emotions is akin to increasing one's palate of emotions. Pandemics bring about incredibly emotional times, and one is likely to experience waves of different emotions. Not having the skills to deal with these emotions when they arise will result in a leader ill-equipped to deal with a crisis.

The second set of skills is the ability to incorporate emotions into one's decision-making. Often leaders are taught to operate with detached rationalism. Still, we know from famous work such as that by Tversky and Kahneman (1974) that logical processes do not purely govern our decision-making. Therefore, leaders should learn to use their emotions as a decision-making aid, as another source of information to test when making a decision (Palmer *et al.*, 2008). Indeed, the failure to engage emotions in decision-making, and not only understand but "feel" how to communicate negative messages, was a differentiator of leadership during COVID-19. The media chastised brands such as Uber and Verge, for the apparent callousness of their redundancy notices, while companies, such as Airbnb, were lauded for their messaging to staff (Forbes, 2020).

The final EI competencies to review are the skills required to understand and motivate (Palmer *et al.*, 2008). Just as leaders will be experiencing a range of emotions, so too will their followers. Effective leadership will be not only recognising the emotions other people are feeling, but more importantly, being able to intervene and to motivate them accordingly.

Given the relationship to other leadership behaviours, EI can be considered the meta-skill for leaders to navigate a crisis. The scientific rigour of EI competencies is not what is essential. Instead, what is important is how the concepts of EI translate into practice. What is important is whether the leader will develop these skills to enhance their capacity to deal with the trial and tribulations that they and their staff, will have to deal with through the pandemic. Evidence from programmes to develop EI skills in leaders, such as GENOS, indicates that leaders can develop EI and that the development leads to positive organisational outcomes. Leaders who demonstrate the various EI competencies demonstrate a greater ability to meet achievement and developmental needs of their subordinates, motivate and inspire others to work towards a common goal, and do more than is expected (Gardner & Stough, 2002; Palmer *et al.*, 2001).

A key to enhancing the functioning of an organisation in a pandemic is the development of leaders that are pandemic-ready. Not being prepared for a pandemic is something that leaders will be given a pass for once. Given that organisations have now experienced a pandemic, the future expectation will be that leaders have the skills to prepare and guide organisations and employees, through the crisis precipitated by the pandemic. Given the lessons learnt from COVID-19, preparations to be more resilient in a crisis will start immediately, and pandemic preparation should now be on all the development plans of leaders. The cost of not being prepared is too high for all, but the most robust company balance sheet to withstand. Unlike the preparation required to strengthen fixed assets and physical systems, the development of leadership skills is the development of soft skills.

The preparation will include, as a critical meta-skill, the deepening of emotional skills to help leaders to help themselves through the crisis as well as the ability to lead others. Organisations will expect leaders to cultivate operational excellence so that the drop in performance due to changes in working practices brought on by the crisis, is minimised. Qualities of authentic leadership will be required so that leaders are trusted and respected. Leaders will also be required to demonstrate creativity and formulate visions, potentially undeveloped skills in their current leadership repertoire.

The development of all the skills discussed in this chapter will take time. Some leaders may already have aspects of each skill area, but it is unlikely that any leaders will have no room to grow in at least one of the five areas discussed. A pandemic may represent one of the ultimate tests for a leader, and the lessons learnt via the COVID-19 pandemic provide a blueprint for the type of skills that leaders need to cultivate in the future to prepare for the next crisis.

# References

Baron, J., & Francois, B. (2020, April 27). A crisis playbook for the family business. *Harvard Business Review*. https://hbr.org/2020/04/a-crisis-playbook-for-family-businesses

Bunker, K. A. (1997). The power of vulnerability in contemporary leadership. *Consulting Psychology Journal: Practice and Research, 49*(2), 122–136.

Burke, C. S., Sims, D. E., Lazzara, E. H., & Salas, E. (2007). Trust in leadership: A multi-level review and integration. *The Leadership Quarterly, 18*(6), 606–632.

Clear, J. (2018). *Atomic habits: An easy & proven way to build good habits & break bad ones.* Penguin.

Companies still not prepared to respond to COVID-19 people and business implications. (2020, March 16). *People Matters.* https://www.peoplemattersglobal.com/article/c-suite/companies-still-not-prepared-to-respond-to-covid-19-people-and-business-implications-25005

Dunford, D., Dale, B., Stylianou, N., Lowther, E., Ahmed, M., & Arenas, I. d. l. T. (2020, April 7). Coronavirus: The world in lockdown in maps and charts. *BBC News.* https://www.bbc.com/news/world-52103747

Englert, P., Seymour, S., & Johnstone, S. (2006). The Development and Application of a three-factor Leadership Model. *New Zealand Journal of Human Resource Management, 6*, 1–23.

EY Global. (2020, March 19). *COVID-19 and pandemic planning: How companies should respond.* https://www.ey.com/en_gl/covid-19/covid-19-and-pandemic-planning--how-companies-should-respond

Gallo, C. (2020, March 21). Marriott's CEO demonstrates truly authentic leadership in a remarkably emotional video. *Forbes.* https://www.forbes.com/sites/carminegallo/2020/03/21/marriotts-ceo-demonstrates-truly-authentic-leadership-in-a-remarkably-emotional-video/#79d9c5691654

Gardner, L., & Stough, C. (2002). Examining the relationship between leadership and emotional intelligence in senior level managers. *Leadership & Organization Development Journal, 23*, 68–78.

Gardner, W. L., Avolio, B. J., Luthans, F., May, D. R., & Walumbwa, F. (2005). "Can you see the real me?" A self-based model of authentic leader and follower development. *The Leadership Quarterly, 16*(3), 343–372.

Hitt, M., Ireland, R. D., & Hoskisson, R. (2012). *Strategic management cases: competitiveness and globalisation.* Cengage Learning.

Horton, R. (2020, March 18). UK failures over Covid-19 will increase death toll, says leading doctor. *The Guardian.* https://www.theguardian.com/society/2020/mar/18/uk-failures-over-covid-19-will-increase-death-toll-says-leading-doctor

House, R. J. (1971). A 1976 theory of path-goal leadership. *Administrative Science Quarterly, 16*, 321–338.

House, R. J., Dorfman, P. W., Javidan, M., Hanges, P. J., & de Luque, M. F. S. (2013). *Strategic leadership across cultures: GLOBE study of CEO leadership behavior and effectiveness in 24 countries.* Sage Publications.

House, R. J., & Shamir, B. (1993). Toward an integration of transformational, charismatic and visionary theories of leadership. In M. Chemmers & R. Ayman (Eds.), *Leadership: Perspectives and research directions* (pp. 81–107). Academic Press.

Hughes, R. L., Ginnett, R. C., & Curphy, G. J. (1999). *Leadership: Enhancing the lessons of experience.* Boston: McGraw-Hill.

Iacurci, G. (2020, May 19). Unemployment is nearing Great Depression levels. Here's how the eras are similar—and different. *CNBC.* https://www.cnbc.com/2020/05/19/unemployment-today-vs-the-great-depression-how-do-the-eras-compare.html

Ireland, R. D., & Hitt, M. (2005). Achieving and maintaining strategic competitiveness in the 21st Century: The role of strategic leadership. *Academy of Management, 19*(4), 63–77.

Jandhyala, S. (2020, March 22). Why your firms' internal processes may determine the business impact of COVID-19. *Singapore Business Review.* https://sbr.com.sg/economy/commentary/why-your-firms-internal-processes-may-determine-business-impact-covid-19

Jiang, M. (2020, April 23). The reason Zoom calls drain your energy. *BBC News.* https://www.bbc.com/worklife/article/20200421-why-zoom-video-chats-are-so-exhausting?utm_source=Nature+Briefing&utm_campaign=d7ac20f928-briefing-dy-20200422&utm_medium=email&utm_term=0_c9dfd39373-d7ac20f928-43709501

Kelly, J. (2020, May 13). Uber lays off 3,500 employees over a Zoom call—The way in which a company downsizes its staff says a lot about the organisation. *Forbes.* https://www.forbes.com/sites/jackkelly/2020/05/13/uber-lays-off-3500-employees-over-a-zoom-call-the-way-in-which-a-company-downsizes-its-staff-says-a-lot-about-the-organization/#192e03807251

Koehn, N. (2020, April 3). Real leaders are forged in a crisis. *Harvard Business Review.* https://hbr.org/2020/04/real-leaders-are-forged-in-crisis

Ladkin, D., & Taylor, S. S. (2010). Enacting the "true self": Towards a theory of embodied authentic leadership. *The Leadership Quarterly, 21*(1), 64–74.

Landy, F. J., & Conte, J. M. (2018). *Work in the 21st century: An introduction to industrial and organisational psychology* (6th ed.). John Wiley & Sons.

Lewis, A., & Clark, J. (2020). Dreams within a dream: Multiple visions and organisational structure. *Journal of Organizational Behavior, 41*(1), 50–76.

McCarthy J. (2020, April 25). Praised For Curbing COVID-19, New Zealand's Leader Eases Country's Strict Lockdown. *NPR.* https://www.npr.org/sections/coronavirus-live-updates/2020/04/25/844720581/praised-for-curbing-covid-19-new-zealands-leader-eases-country-s-strict-lockdown

Marr, B. (2020, March 17). How the COVID-19 pandemic is fast-tracking digital transformation in companies. *Forbes.* https://www.forbes.com/sites/bernardmarr/2020/03/17/how-the-covid-19-pandemic-is-fast-tracking-digital-transformation-in-companies/#1b9ae465a8ee

Ministry of Manpower. (2020). *Advisory on safe distancing measures at the workplace.* https://www.mom.gov.sg/covid-19/advisory-on-safe-distancing-measures

Newport, C. (2016). *Deep work: Rules for focused success in a distracted world.* Hachette UK.

Newport, C. (2017, March 13). *Yuval Harari works less than you.* Study Hacks. https://www.calnewport.com/blog/2017/03/13/yuval-harari-works-less-than-you/

Nielson, K. (2020, May 4). Managing workplace survivor syndrome after redundancies. *HRM.* https://www.hrmonline.com.au/covid-19/managing-workplace-survivor-syndrome-redundancies/

Nienaber, A. M., Hofeditz, M., & Romeike, P. D. (2015). Vulnerability and trust in leader-follower relationships. *Personnel Review, 44*(4), 567–591.

Palmer, B. R., Gignac, G. E., Ekermans, G., & Stough, C. (2008). A comprehensive framework for emotional intelligence. In R. Emmerling, M. K. Mandal, & V. K. Shanwal (Eds.), *Emotional intelligence: Theoretical & cultural perspectives* (pp. 17–38). Nova Science Publishing.

Palmer, B., Walls, M., Burgess, Z., & Stough, C. (2001). Emotional intelligence and effective leadership. *Leadership & Organization Development Journal, 22,* 5–10.

Paulus, P. (2000). Groups, teams, and creativity: The creative potential of idea-generating groups. *Applied Psychology, 49*(2), 237–262.

Podsakoff, N. P., Blume, B., Whiting, S., & Podsakoff, P. (2009). Individual- and organisational-level consequences of organisational citizenship behaviors: A meta-analysis. *Journal of Applied Psychology, 94,* 122–141.

Pulakos, E. D., Arad, S., Donovan, M. A., & Plamondon, K. E. (2000). Adaptability in the workplace: Development of a taxonomy of adaptive performance. *Journal of Applied Psychology, 85*(4), 612–624.

Reeves, M., & Fuller, J. (2020, April 10). We need imagination now more than ever. *Harvard Business Review*. https://hbr.org/2020/04/we-need-imagination-now-more-than-ever

Riley, C. (2020, May 7). The UK economy is heading for its worst crash in 300 years. *CNN Business*. https://edition.cnn.com/2020/05/07/economy/uk-economy-bank-of-england/index.html

Teo, W. L., Lee, M., & Lim, W. S. (2017). The relational activation of resilience model: How leadership activates resilience in an organisational crisis. *Journal of Contingencies and Crisis Management, 25*(3), 136–147.

The Coronavirus pandemic is a failure of leadership—not intelligence (2020, April 3). *Small Wars Journal*. https://smallwarsjournal.com/jrnl/art/coronavirus-pandemic-failure-leadership-not-intelligence

Tversky, A., & Kahneman, D. (1974). Judgment under uncertainty: Heuristics and biases. *Science, 185*, 1,124–1,131.

Worley, C. G., & Jules, C. (2020 In Press). COVID-19's uncomfortable revelations about agile and sustainable organisations in a VUCA World. *Journal of Applied Behavioral Science*, 1–5. https://doi.org/10.1177/0021886320936263

Zeidner, M., Matthews, G. M., & Roberts, R. (2001). Slow down, you move too fast: Emotional intelligence remains an "elusive" intelligence. *Emotions, 1*, 265–275.

Zeidner, M., Matthews, G., & Roberts, R. (2004). "Emotional intelligence in the workplace: A critical review". *Applied Psychology: An International Review, 53*, 371–399.

# Chapter 14

# Sustaining Team Morale Amidst a Pandemic: Lessons from COVID-19

Minzheng Hou

## Introduction

COVID-19 has led to sustained health emergencies across the world. Efforts to combat, contain, and mitigate the spread of the virus have been complex and prolonged, with public service officers—e.g., healthcare workers, law enforcers, contact tracers—working tirelessly for months on end (Cheong, 2020). For many of these officers, especially those deployed at the frontlines (e.g., hospitals, community care facilities, quarantine facilities), these operations may be particularly daunting. Safety risks are high given the potential for infection. The high volume of patients and uncertain medical trajectory of the virus render a fast-paced and dynamic operating environment unavoidable. Moreover, given the relatively rare occurrence of such a potent disease outbreak, many officers could have been deployed for duties of such nature for the first time.

Consequently, emotional responses like fear and anxiety may ensue. This is coupled with harsh work environments (brought about by the prolonged nature of the operations leading to fatigue), the experience of grief after observing deaths, the reduced team cohesion due to disruptive safe distancing measures requiring teams to segregate themselves and reduce physical interactions. Together, these stressors may cause officers to lose confidence in their abilities to fulfil their duties, or even experience a fatalistic outlook towards the situation (Goh, 2020).

197

Inevitably, these elements inherent in frontline COVID-19 operations have a very real, detrimental impact on frontliners' morale, and hence operational effectiveness. As morale is a crucial ingredient in ensuring commitment, motivation, and perseverance in the face of difficulty (Jones *et al.*, 2012; Ryan & Deci, 2000), cultivating high morale is critical in engendering within our officers the will and tenacity to persist amidst challenges in these high-stress and high-risk operations.

The present chapter provides a brief overview of what morale is, and provides recommendations on what leaders can do to sustain high team morale during operations such as those seen in the COVID-19 pandemic.

## Understanding Morale

Morale has long been recognised as a vital ingredient for operational success. As a fuzzy concept, however, definitions of morale in the literature remain vague, with various researchers diverging in their assessment on what specifically constitutes morale. For example, Britt and Dickinson (2006) referred to morale as a positive motivational state related to superior performance under stress, adaptive responding to operational demands, and positive job attitudes. Manning (1991) described morale as the sense of enthusiasm and persistence that characterise teams when striving towards their mission objectives. González-Romá and colleagues (2006) further identified dedication and vigour as a reflection of morale.

Notwithstanding these diverging theoretical perspectives, researchers remain unanimous in their acknowledgement of the significant impact that morale has on a team's motivation, cohesion, and operational effectiveness (Motowidlo & Borman, 1978; van Boxmeer *et al.*, 2010). Indeed, teams with high morale reap substantial benefits. For instance, team members with high morale enjoy greater performance and stronger commitment to the organisation (Alonso & Lewis, 2001). They are also more likely to exhibit greater organisational citizenship behaviours (i.e., going above and beyond their scope of duty to help their group), and have a greater sense of belonging and ownership towards their work (Valsania *et al.*, 2012). These are crucial ingredients that help sustain a team's effectiveness, and ensure that the team achieves its objectives.

Moreover, sustaining high morale is essential not only during peacetime but more importantly, during a crisis when everyone must come together, pull their weight, and overcome significant challenges. To achieve such a desirable and optimal state in a team during crisis operations, leaders in government agencies must endeavour to set the necessary conditions for morale to be sustained even under highly stressful environments. This chapter will cover five recommendations to do so.

## Recommendation #1: Appeal to Core Values and Higher-Order Aspects

One key enabler to enhance morale is to appeal to higher-order core values and rationale during communications with the team. This means providing teams with a narrative on why they are doing what they are doing, and illustrating the foundational basis on which their actions ought to be guided (Jong, 2017). Doing so provides teams with a clear sense of meaning and purpose, allows individuals to transcend themselves, and to act in service of the wider community.

Importantly, leaders should emphasise core values that are of a self-transcendental nature (e.g., honour to one's country, selfless service). Indeed, psychological research has provided evidence that self-transcendence can be a particularly important factor in engendering motivation towards a shared objective (Yeager *et al.*, 2014). Specifically, cultivating a self-transcendental purpose serves as a basis for teams to feel inspired towards something greater than themselves (Hou & Thenarianto, 2020). It also allows individuals to keep their sights onto something higher, and thus aids in fostering an unwavering fighting spirit to overcome adversities.

In this regard, self-transcendental organisational core values such as honour, courage, and loyalty, serve as a useful vision for team members to keep in sight. They serve as a psychological compass to guide behaviour and responses to setback. Notably, they are both an end in and of themselves (i.e., they illuminate the self-transcendental objectives of the teams' actions), as well as a means to the end (i.e., they describe how teams ought to carry themselves at all times) (Eccles & Wigfield, 2002; Mayfield *et al.*, 2015). In other words, team members deployed for operations should recognise that core values form the basis of why they do what they do, and how they ought to go about doing them.

During a crisis such as COVID-19, team members should recognise that they are not merely individuals working for self-interest, but are serving something larger than themselves. Specifically, leaders should emphasise the crucial role of their teams in safeguarding Singapore's internal safety and security, highlighting the respective organisation's core values in rallying their officers. Such messages from leaders, including via command briefings in person or through email, may articulate that challenging times, such as these, are precisely when officers ought to embody and act in accordance with organisational core values.

Furthermore, to unite teams towards a shared vision, leaders may talk in terms of a common destiny for all when addressing teams. For example, phrases such as "This is about us getting through this crisis together", "This crisis affects all of us" may be considered. It is also important to emphasise the common objective of securing Singapore's future together, such as "We all have a duty to Singapore, to ensure her safety and security". Doing so is particularly important given that the tasks assigned to team members may differ; the course of daily operations for some may be repetitive or dynamic, at the frontlines or at back-end support. It is, therefore, crucial to ensure that every team member recognises the same, common mission objective despite their differing roles.

## Recommendation #2: Foster an Unwavering Team Spirit

During the COVID-19 pandemic, frontline teams work tirelessly around the clock for prolonged periods of time. The extended nature of the pandemic simply means that they have to continue working endlessly till a sustainable end-state can be achieved. From sustaining prolonged shift-work, to working extended hours and holding concurrent duties, many team members are invariably stretched and fatigued. However, what keeps teams going—and indeed, what makes a team—is knowing that team members have each other's back (Bounds, 2020).

As teamwork and team cohesiveness are vital components of morale (Britt & Dickinson, 2006), leaders play an indispensable role in creating the conditions and norms necessary for team cohesion. In particular, teams need to recognise that a strong sense of team spirit is not something that a team naturally possesses (or not), but rather, is a choice that every individual team member must make.

In other words, every team member has the responsibility to decide to be a team member, and to support one another at all times. In this regard, it is a leader's core responsibility to foster such consciousness among their team. Leaders, in their communication with the team, should aim to establish supportive behaviour that makes teamwork the norm. This entails leaders constantly encouraging their team to support one another in any way they can. For example, using team-based narratives ("we are in this together"), languages (using "we"), and images (showing teams working together) in briefings and emails. In addition, leaders can actively ask that team members cover each other's duties where needed, demonstrate care and concern for one another, and encourage one another to persevere.

To further entrench a shared consciousness of working together as one, leaders should also personally walk the ground to provide leadership presence to rally their people (Gal & Manning, 1987). Leadership presence—i.e., a willingness to "get their hands dirty"—is crucial not only in demonstrating leadership by example, but in conveying a sense of togetherness and positive connection with one's leader. Indeed, the failure of leaders to be with their people through thick and thin only serves to alienate the leader from the team and threatens team members' confidence and trust in their leader (Gal & Manning, 1987).

## Recommendation #3: Recognise Each Other's Sacrifice

Setbacks and frustrations are inevitable in the course of daily operations. Especially within a dynamic and fast-paced operating environment, it is natural at times for emotions to run high and stress to feel overbearing. In these situations, it may be easy for some to feel overwhelmed, burned out, or even despair. Amidst the constant hustle, leaders may neglect that very often, a simple positive affirmation can go a long way in warming hearts, providing meaning and assurance, and sustaining commitment.

Positive affirmation includes praise for good work done, recognition of sacrifices put in, and appreciating each other's efforts. It allows people to celebrate small successes along the way, breaking down seemingly insurmountable tasks into smaller, manageable steps. The provision of such a sense of progression through one's striving is indeed an important element in sustaining motivation, especially when it comes to one's longer-term or larger scale endeavours (Koestner *et al.*, 2008; Moskowitz & Grant, 2009), such as the prolonged battle against COVID-19. In other words, it is important that leaders do not neglect celebrating small successes with their teams along the way. These include praising team members' effort and hard work promptly, including even small achievements, or explicitly appreciating efforts and sacrifices in briefings and emails. These small acts of warmth and kindness may well provide just that extra bit of morale boost, enabling individuals to persevere in their endeavours.

Furthermore, cultivating a positive and encouraging work environment is key to overcoming the tendency for one to slip into a "critical" mode during these operations. After all, amidst the demanding and risky operating environment, it may be easy for one to focus almost exclusively on critiquing negative behaviour or faults due to an emphasis on preventing mistakes, and thereby overlook the important role of positive feedback in promoting positive behaviour (Henley & DiGennaro Reed, 2015).

Indeed, while the intention to avoid errors is crucial in high stakes environments, it is also important for leaders to bear in mind the unintended consequences of cultivating an atmosphere of excessive fear in an already stressful period. As such, it may be equally important for leaders to leverage on positive words of encouragement and affirmation to sustain team members' morale in these challenging times.

## Recommendation #4: Create Psychologically Safe Spaces

Through the course of their duty, team members will no doubt have feedback and concerns pertaining to the operations in which they are involved. This is to be expected, given that individuals have different risk appetites, coping strategies, and even operational endurance (Dewe *et al.*, 1993). As such, it is important for the leaders to create psychologically safe spaces where members feel comfortable to voice their feedback, raise reservations, or even contribute suggestions (Kahn, 1990). Specifically, this entails leadership emphasis at all levels on the value of feedback (especially coming from those engaged in the frontlines who are most at risk), and efforts to establish open communication channels. Ensuring that members' concerns are promptly being heard and acted upon provides the assurance that the organisation cares about them.

In addition, given the rapidly evolving ground situation, these measures to create psychologically safe spaces not only serve to facilitate adaptive and dynamic operational responses, but can also strengthen commitment and motivation towards serving the organisation as one's sense of ownership is enhanced (Allen & Meyer, 1990). Furthermore, it will be important for leaders to closely monitor the fluctuations in psychological states (e.g., anxiety, fear, stress, fatigue levels) of officers and spare no effort in addressing them promptly. The deployment of para-counsellors to keep a lookout for and provide a listening ear to fellow officers can enhance the creation of a psychologically safe space for officers. Close monitoring of psychological states through pulse surveys or observations can allow leaders to take timely steps to safeguard officers' psychological readiness.

## Recommendation #5: Provide Sufficient Safeguards for Team Members

Finally, in the course of performing their duties, not only do officers' psychological well-being need to be safeguarded, their physical well-being too must also be protected. In other words, leaders must endeavour to provide both a tangible and intangible sense of safety for their teams. Indeed, healthcare practitioners had extensively displayed concerns about protecting themselves, their families, and their staff from the virus during the SARS outbreak in 2003 (Wong *et al.*, 2004). Providing officers with a sense of being tangibly protected by the organisation thus allows them to perform their duties confidently with a peace of mind.

In this regard, team members need to know that sufficient safeguards are/will be put in place to protect the safety and welfare of themselves and their loved ones. For example, the provision of personal protective equipment and the coverage of healthcare-related costs for both officers and their families are among some important "hygiene" issues that provide a sense of tangible security.

Other measures to safeguard the welfare of officers may include conducive rest points, such as those offering some privacy away from the public and allowing officers to decompress from the stress of their duties. Leaders can also consider setting up alternate rest sites for officers who do not wish to proceed home after their duties for fear of infecting their loved ones, and ensuring adequate provisions for basic needs such as food and transport. These measures are aimed at ensuring that team members' basic needs and concerns are met, so as to provide them with a peace of mind in delivering operational effectiveness.

# Conclusion

In the various operations required during a pandemic, sustaining high morale is key to ensuring operational effectiveness and mission success. This chapter has highlighted how the nature of a prolonged pandemic may lead to team morale being compromised, given the elements present in various operational duties. These elements include the prolonged nature of the operations leading to fatigue, the experience of grief after observing deaths, the reduced team cohesion due to disruptive safe distancing measures requiring teams to segregate themselves and reduce physical interactions. Those deployed at the frontlines may be especially affected by these elements.

In response, this chapter outlines five recommendations that team leaders should bear in mind during operational planning. First, team leaders must strive to sustain high morale by appealing to core values and higher-order aspects (e.g., the Nation in need) to provide a sense of purpose in team members across functions and level. In other words, officers should be motivated to unite and transcend the self in service of the larger good. Second, team leaders have an indispensable role to play in cultivating the norms and behaviours necessary for team cohesion, a crucial component of morale. Specifically, team leaders need to recognise that teamwork is a choice, and to foster positive norms of teamwork by emphasising to team members to support one another at all times. Third, leaders should not neglect to celebrate small successes along the way, and to provide positive affirmation (e.g., recognition of effort and sacrifice) to their team members to provide that extra morale boost. Fourth, it is important for leaders to create psychologically safe spaces for the raising of feedback and concerns. Helping officers feel heard is crucial in fostering a sense of belonging and ownership in their work. It is also crucial to monitor fluctuating levels of psychological responses (e.g., anxiety, stress) closely in order to provide timely assistance. Finally, sufficient tangible safeguards should also be provided for officers to address their basic needs; officers' welfare must be protected before they can perform their duties with a peace of mind.

# References

Allen, N. J., & Meyer, J. P. (1990). The measurement and antecedents of affective, continuance and normative commitment to the organisation. *Journal of Occupational Psychology, 63*(1), 1–18. https://doi.org/10.1111/j.2044-8325.1990.tb00506.x

Alonso, P., & Lewis, G. B. (2001). Public service motivation and job performance: Evidence from the federal sector. *The American Review of Public Administration, 31*(4), 363–380. https://doi.org/10.1177/02750740122064992

Bounds, A. (2020, April, 19). Harnessing the power of teamwork to tackle coronavirus. *Financial Times.* https://www.ft.com/content/19920214-703c-11ea-89df-41bea055720b

Britt, T. W., & Dickinson, J. M. (2006). Morale during military operations: A positive psychology approach. In T. W. Britt., C. A. Castro., & A. B. Adler (Eds.), *Military life: The psychology of serving in peace and combat: Vol. 1. Military performance* (pp. 157–184). Westport, CT: Praeger Security International.

Cheong, D. (2020, February 2). Wuhan virus: Singapore must prepare for battle over long haul, says Chan Chun Sing. *The Straits Times.* https://www.straitstimes.com/singapore/wuhan-virus-singapore-must-prepare-for-battle-over-long-haul-says-chan-chun-sing

Dewe, P., Cox, T., & Ferguson, E. (1993). Individual strategies for coping with stress at work: A review. *Work & Stress, 7*(1), 5–15. https://doi.org/10.1080/02678379308257046

Eccles, J. S., & Wigfield, A. (2002). Motivational beliefs, values, and goals. *Annual Review of Psychology, 53*(1), 109–132. https://doi.org/10.1146/annurev.psych.53.100901.135153

Gal, R., & Manning, F. J. (1987). Morale and its components: A cross-national comparison. *Journal of Applied Social Psychology, 17*(4), 369–391. https://doi.org/10.1111/j.1559-1816.1987.tb00319.x

Goh, C. T. (2020, May 3). COVID-19: Guarding against burnout, compassion fatigue and trauma in frontline healthcare workers. *Channel NewsAsia.* https://www.channelnewsasia.com/news/singapore/covid-19-guarding-against-burnout-trauma-ttsh-ncid-frontline-12669280

González-Romá, V., Schaufeli, W. B., Bakker, A. B., & Lloret, S. (2006). Burnout and work engagement: Independent factors or opposite poles? *Journal of Vocational Behavior, 68*(1), 165–174. https://doi.org/10.1016/j.jvb.2005.01.003

Henley, A. J., & DiGennaro Reed, F. D. (2015). Should you order the feedback sandwich? Efficacy of feedback sequence and timing. *Journal of Organizational Behavior Management, 35*(3–4), 321–335. https://doi.org/10.1080/01608061.2015.1093057

Hou, M., & Thenarianto, J. J. (2020). Inspirational leadership: How does one inspire another? *HTBSC Brief Research Report 20/2020.* Singapore: Home Team Behavioural Sciences Centre.

Jones, N., Seddon, R., Fear, N. T., McAllister, P., Wessely, S., & Greenberg, N. (2012). Leadership, cohesion, morale, and the mental health of UK Armed Forces in Afghanistan. *Psychiatry: Interpersonal and Biological Processes, 75*(1), 49–59. https://doi.org/10.1521/psyc.2012.75.1.49

Jong, W. (2017). Meaning making by public leaders in times of crisis: An assessment. *Public Relations Review*, *43*(5), 1,025–1,035. https://doi.org/10.1016/j.pubrev.2017.09.003

Kahn, W. A. (1990). Psychological conditions of personal engagement and disengagement at work. *The Academy of Management Journal*, *33*(4), 692–724. https://doi.org/10.5465/256287

Koestner, R., Otis, N., Powers, T. A., Pelletier, L., & Gagnon, H. (2008). Autonomous motivation, controlled motivation, and goal progress. *Journal of Personality*, *76*(5), 1,201–1,230. https://doi.org/10.1111/j.1467-6494.2008.00519.x

Manning, F. J. (1991). Morale, cohesion, and esprit de corps. In Gal, R. & Mangelsdorff, A. D. (Eds.), *Handbook of Military Psychology* (pp. 453–470). Chichester: John Wiley & Sons Ltd.

Mayfield, J., Mayfield, M., & Sharbrough, W. C. (2015). Strategic vision and values in top leaders' communications: Motivating language at a higher level. *International Journal of Business Communication*, *52*(1), 97–121. https://doi.org/10.1177/2329488414560282

Moskowitz, G. B., & Grant, H. (Eds.). (2009). *The psychology of goals*. New York, NY: Guilford Press.

Motowidlo, S. J., & Borman, W. C. (1978). Relationships between military morale, motivation, satisfaction, and unit effectiveness. *Journal of Applied Psychology*, *63*(1), 47–52. https://doi.org/10.1037/0021-9010.63.1.47

Ryan, R. M., & Deci, E. L. (2000). Self-determination theory and the facilitation of intrinsic motivation, social development, and well-being. *American Psychologist*, *55*(1), 68–78. https://doi.org/10.1037//0003-066X.55.1.68

Valsania, S. E., Moriano León, J. A., Alonso, F. M., & Cantisano, G. T. (2012). Authentic leadership and its effect on employees' organisational citizenship behaviors. *Psicothema*, *24*(4), 561–566. https://psycnet.apa.org/record/2012-28458-009

van Boxmeer, L. E. L. M., Verwijs, C., Euwema, M., & van Dalenberg, S. (2010). *Assessing morale and psychological distress during modern military operations*. Paper presented at the 52nd Conference of the International Military Testing Association, 27 September–1 October, Lucerne, Switzerland.

Wong, W. C. W., Lee, A., Tsang, K. K., & Wong, S. Y. S. (2004). How did general practitioners protect themselves, their family, and staff during the SARS epidemic in Hong Kong? *Journal of Epidemiology and Community Health*, *58*(3), 180–185. https://doi.org/10.1136/jech.2003.015594

Yeager, D. S., Henderson, M. D., Paunesku, D., Walton, G. M., D'Mello, S., Spitzer, B. J., & Duckworth, A. L. (2014). Boring but important: A self-transcendent purpose for learning fosters academic self-regulation. *Journal of Personality and Social Psychology*, *107*(4), 559–580. https://doi.org/10.1037/a0037637

# Chapter 15

# Telecommuting During a Pandemic: Tips for Parents and Caregivers of the Elderly

Vivian Seah, John Yu, and Whistine Chai

## Introduction

"Work from Home", or WFH, has become a ubiquitous term in the second quarter of 2020 throughout the globe. Once viewed as a luxury or even a hassle by some, it has become a necessity for the workforce at large to continue their operations during social distancing and lockdown measures imposed by countries during the COVID-19 pandemic. This sudden transition to telecommuting has undoubtedly interrupted the traditional paradigm of work for many who were forced to WFH. From retail to education sectors to judicial hearings, digital technologies have been rapidly adopted to enable remote interactions and continuation of essential services (Bowcott, 2020; Li & Lalani, 2020; Wahba, 2020).

Amidst the whirlwind of change in industries and organisations, a significant factor that should not be neglected is the impact of telecommuting on the lives of new telecommuters. Some converts have viewed telecommuting as a silver lining during the pandemic; they argued that there is more time available for individual pursuits and family commitments. At the same time, anecdotal reports and commentaries have surfaced the plight of some WFH employees who have experienced higher levels of stress and anxiety, decrease in productivity, and decline in mental health and emotional regulation (Murphy, 2020; Rosenbaum,

2020; Teo, 2020). Telecommuting might turn out to be a double-edged sword, and it is vital to understand and support workers who may be struggling with such arrangements in the long run.

More specifically, two categories of workers might experience more strain with telecommuting than others: (1) parents with younger children, and (2) caregivers of the elderly. Amidst the pandemic, schools, childcare centres and services, as well as eldercare facilities have been temporarily closed in many countries, and outdoor mobility is severely restricted by mandatory COVID-19 measures. Parents and caregivers now find it increasingly challenging, at times even overwhelming, to balance work with family commitments over a prolonged period (O'Donnell, 2020). With competing demands from work and family co-occurring, work–family conflicts may arise and escalate if not handled properly, resulting in greater psychological stress and strained relationships (Young, 2020).

Therefore, this chapter explores how WFH employees can better cope with telecommuting and caring for children and the elderly at the same time. Based on research and best practices proposed by worldwide experts, this chapter will offer five tips on how to cope with family commitments while working from home.

# Tip #1: Establish Boundaries And Family Schedules

## *Establish Clear Boundaries between Professional and Family Roles*

With prolonged WFH arrangements, one's personal and private space for respite may inadvertently be fused with one's workplace. This arrangement may encourage cross-role disruptions (e.g., having to switch between parenting or caregiving role and work role). Boundaries between work and personal roles can become highly intertwined, with one being unable to psychologically disengage one role from another. This may foster heightened anxiety, role confusion, work–life conflict, and poorer productivity (Ashforth *et al.*, 2000).

It is thus important to ensure the segmentation of different roles by establishing clear physical boundaries while telecommuting. This could be done in several ways—e.g., demarcating a designated workspace, closing the door to the workstation, and being dressed in work attire during stipulated office hours even in the comfort of home. These physical changes could allow one to psychologically attune to their salient role at the stipulated time—e.g., work during office hours (Salazar, 2001). It is also vital to inculcate a routine that signals a workday has ended, for instance, by shutting down and keeping away one's work laptop, or going for a short walk to disengage from work and transit into one's personal role (Terrell, 2020).

In addition, it is beneficial to form rules and boundaries with household members to balance their expectations on when their parents and caregivers are available for them. Parents could explain to their children that as long as they are working during certain times of the day, they will not be able to engage in playtime or activities with them. Employees who are caring for elderly members may need to explain to them that working from home is not a substitute for full-time care as the elderly may not be familiar to the idea of WFH (Arbaje, 2020). Situations that warrant interruption to these rules should be discussed with family members to align their understanding and expectations on when the boundaries can be breached.

## *Plan Family Schedules That Best Cater to Everyone*

It may be challenging for some to stipulate clear boundaries between work and family life, especially for those who have to care for the daily needs and activities (e.g., meals, exercises, medication) of their children or elderly parents. One could work around this issue by planning schedules and establishing routines that best complement the needs of all family members. This would minimise abrupt changes to the schedule and encourage all to commit to the family schedule. Schedules and routines that are holistically tailored to one's family can help to inject structure at home and help telecommuters feel in control, reducing anxiety and work–family conflict (Ehmke, 2020).

For instance, parents could work on a rotational basis if they are both telecommuting and their children require babysitting—it may be helpful to assign "shift work", in which one parent takes the first parenting shift from 8 a.m. to 1 p.m., while the other takes the second shift from 1 p.m. to 6 p.m. This routine allows one parent to work in full concentration without guilt while their spouse cares for the child. Such arrangements will be especially useful for parents with young children who require constant care or supervision of their school work. For those caring for the elderly, one might need to consider whether their telecommuting schedule might overlap with the elderly's essential activities. For example, it may be helpful to refrain from scheduling a video conference call during mealtimes as the elderly may require assistance to eat, or they might look forward to having meals together.

Although routines and schedules can help one to better cope with telecommuting during a pandemic, there should be flexibility in adapting to changes in schedules than enforce a schedule that does not seem to fit well. Being flexible to changes in schedule may be helpful as research has found that psychological flexibility is associated with a decrease in stress levels and an increase in well-being (Wersebe *et al.*, 2018). There is no "one-size-fits-all" schedule, and it may take days, weeks, or even months to experiment and fine-tune a schedule that best fits one's family.

### *Set Actionable and Practical Goals*

The new norm of telecommuting may prove to be a struggle for those who are new to it. Setting daily goals for tasks could help one to cope with working in a new environment while remaining productive. One way is to adopt the Pomodoro technique to maximise productivity and get more work done within a shorter span of time. The Pomodoro technique could consist of the following steps (Cirillo, 2006):

1. Set a work goal or a task to be done.
2. Set the timer for an undisturbed period of time—e.g., 25 minutes.
3. Work on the task with full concentration until the timer rings—i.e., this is considered one "Pomodoro".
4. Take a short five minutes break.
5. Consider repeating steps 1 to 4, and take a longer break after four cycles of Pomodoro.

## Tip #2: Communicate more Rather than Less

### *Seek to Understand and Acknowledge Fears and Worries Faced by Children*

Living amidst a prolonged pandemic would be a new experience for families with children as children tend to respond to stress in different ways—some may be open to talking about it, while others may "call for help" through behavioural indicators (Centers for Disease Control and Prevention, 2020a). These include sudden changes in behaviour such as excessive crying or irritation in children, excessive worry or sadness, irritability, unexplained headaches or physical symptoms, avoidance of previously enjoyable activities, and when the child is clinging to their parents more than usual (Centers for Disease Control and Prevention, 2020a). When such sudden behavioural changes are observed in a child, it is good to address them immediately by asking open-ended questions (i.e., what, why, who, where, and how questions), in order to invite children to talk about their worries and concerns (Waite *et al.*, 2020). It is important not to minimise or dismiss children's worries and change in behaviour, but instead, provide the assurance that this disruption in routine would be temporary.

## *Exchange Honest and Appropriate Information with Family*

Communication could also help family members to be more understanding to a telecommuting employee at home. This could be done by providing honest and appropriate information about the pandemic to help regulate family members' and one's own emotions, while living and working together at home during a lockdown. Giving family members the time and space to ask questions is also helpful to alleviate anxiety.

Telecommuting parents could provide their children with clear, honest, and age-appropriate information about COVID-19. Guidelines published by the World Health Organisation (2020a) highlights that such information on the disease and situation can help children cope with the stress and confusion of being cooped up at home during this pandemic. Clearly explaining the rationale for staying indoors and the importance of adhering to the restriction could help children understand and comply with the plans and new routine. There are guidelines (Centers for Disease Control and Prevention, 2020b; National Association of School Psychologists, 2020) and online resources for parents to explain COVID-19 to their children according to their level of understanding.

On the other hand, telecommuting employees with elderly parents could engage in frequent conversations about their welfare. These deliberate conversations can be done periodically to inform the elderly on the new measures implemented, find out about their routines and how they have been interrupted, devise a plan to manage their lifestyle, and steps to take when they are feeling unwell. This can reduce any misunderstandings and lower the stress of living with uncertainties.

### *Set Reasonable Expectations with Co-Workers*

Some employees may find themselves struggling to meet deadlines while juggling family and work commitments. One way to manage this better is to be transparent about one's current home situation with their supervisors and co-workers. Open communication will provide colleagues a clearer picture of one's situation and challenges, and this might help them be more empathetic if one needs to step away from a call or meeting for urgent family matters (O'Donnell, 2020). In addition, making known of these compulsory caregiving duties may help supervisors and co-workers manage their expectations of one's work outputs during the period of WFH.

## Tip #3: Stay Connected with Technology

### *Leverage on Technology for Meaningful Social Interaction*

Telecommuting parents should note that even with social distancing measures in place, peer relationships and social connection are still important in their children's emotional, social, and cognitive development. Research suggests that children with poor peer relationships may suffer from emotional and social adjustment in adolescence, and therefore it is vital to create or retain opportunities for them to meaningfully interact with their peers (Shin *et al.*, 2016). With vast improvements in technology, play dates and hanging out with peers can take place virtually—through video conference sites and applications such as WhatsApp, Skype, Zoom, Google Hangouts, etc. More interestingly, "virtual babysitting" sessions have been favoured during the COVID-19 pandemic lockdown (Elsesser, 2020). Scheduling a virtual babysitting session with extended family members could free up time for telecommuting parents to prepare a meal or simply take a breather from work and parenting.

For telecommuting caregivers of the elderly, it is beneficial for the elderly not to miss out on staying connected with others, even though they may not be savvy in navigating electronic devices. A study on the SARS pandemic in Hong Kong found that having a sense of community-connectedness was a key factor in increasing psychological resilience and well-being during the crisis (Lau *et al.*, 2008). Families and friends who do not have face-to-face contact with the elderly are therefore encouraged to maintain routine conversations via calls or video conferencing. This practice of keeping in touch and supporting them can help to lift their spirits. One could demonstrate and teach the elderly to make video calls to others through their mobile applications, and encourage them to master the use of simple online messaging and video conferencing applications to stay in touch with their family and friends. It may also be helpful for caregivers to help the elderly compile a list of important contacts that they can approach for social interactions whenever the need arises. Compiling this list can reassure them that a diversity of help is merely a phone call away. It can include contacts of other family members, relatives, close friends, and organisations offering counselling and social support services. With these additional sources of support within reach, they may become less reliant on their caregivers, especially while they are working.

## *Harness Technology as a Self-Learning Tool*

Technology could be a lifesaver for telecommuting parents who have to keep their children occupied in the day. It is understandable that parents may worry about giving their children too much screen time for fear of "electronic device dependency". However, when technology is effectively used, children will understand that electronic devices are not just for entertainment, but also serve as important tools for learning (McCombs, 2010). The key is to use digital media strategically—by setting age-appropriate usage quota and promoting the use of electronic devices for educational purposes. Limiting screen time would also be useful in reminding children about the usage quota and yield better cooperation in surrendering the devices when it is time to do so. According to guidelines by the American Academy of Pediatrics (Radesky, 2016), it is advised that screen time should be limited to one hour a day of high-quality content for children who are two to five years old, and no more than two hours of recreational screen time for children above five years old. It is also highlighted that parents could develop a Family Media Plan[1] that highlights screen-free zones and times—e.g., bedrooms, mealtimes, parent–child playtimes, and prior to bedtime (Moreno, 2016).

### *Technology Affords Continual Access to Religious Support*

Religious support has been shown to be one of the key factors in strengthening psychological resilience and helping people tide through a crisis (Foy *et al.*, 2011). Therefore, access to religious support should not be halted during a lockdown. Fortunately, religious groups around the world have continued to support one another through virtual means such as convening online services, and faith-based sharing (Heilweil, 2020). Elderly who feel cut off from their religious groups could attend the online services and outreach efforts with their caregivers to ensure that they remain connected and receive spiritual support from their religious leaders.

## Tip #4: Inject Fun and Keep Active

### *Inject Fun in Mundanities*

Humour has been shown to be an effective coping mechanism in difficult and stressful situations, even during crises (Maxwell, 2003). Therefore, one could inject fun into daily chores and family activities even while telecommuting.

For instance, telecommuting parents could make household chores fun for their children by imbuing them with creative titles such that they become a whole new subject or valued accomplishment—e.g., Honours in Laundry, Masters in Vacuuming, Fine Arts in Food Scooping. This fresh perspective might spur children to help out with such chores so as to be lauded with these achievements, while parents can take a breather. Household chores training could be conducted for children over the weekend as a family activity, and children could be given the opportunity

---

[1]An interactive Family Media Plan was introduced by the American Academy of Paediatrics to help families plan for children screen time and prioritise daily activities. It can be accessed on www.HealthyChildren.org/MediaUsePlan.

to "flaunt their skills" on the weekdays while the telecommuting parent focuses on work commitments. Other fun ideas include singing with the children or the elderly as music has been found to reduce stress and improve mood (Collingwood, 2018). The whole idea is about having fun and staying sane and safe at home during a pandemic lockdown.

### *Stay Physically and Mentally Active*

Keeping active is one way to reduce boredom and negative or anxious thoughts, as well as to provide physiological and psychological benefits while being cooped up at home. Avoiding inactivity at home not only benefits health (Paddock, 2018), but also reduces the likelihood of one interrupting WFH members. One recommendation would be to engage in physical activities such as simple home workouts, as exercise promotes the release of endorphins—a hormone that increases positive moods and alleviates anxiety (Craft & Perna, 2004).

Besides physical activity, one could engage in cognitive activities such as interactive and cognitively-stimulating games that are available online and/or on mobile applications. This may enable everyone in the family, particularly the elderly, to stay mentally engaged during their free time. Other less strenuous home-based activities that can keep the mind active and involve the entire family include board games, indoor gardening, craft-making, organising and decluttering the house, and reminiscing past memories through old photos and mementoes. It is useful to remain curious and open to new activities that can involve the children or entire family amidst this difficult situation.

## Tip #5: Take Care of Your Own Physical and Mental Wellbeing

As mentioned above, it is normal to feel increased levels of stress and anxiety while telecommuting. There is, therefore, a need to be self-aware of one's stress level and to focus on the most important work on hand, instead of pushing oneself over the limit. All these could reduce the chances of WFH employees becoming too overwhelmed and/or experiencing burnout (Giurge & Bohns, 2020).

Furthermore, it is important that telecommuting employees can set aside some time and space for their personal, uninterrupted "me-time" to unwind and do something they enjoy. The World Health Organisation (2020b) recommends the vital need to have sufficient rest, nutrition, physical activity, social connection, and personal time in order to re-energise oneself and avoid burnout. It is also essential not to feel guilty over this me-time, but to treat this short break as a well-deserved rest and reward. If needed, professional help and advice could also be sought as there have been helplines (e.g., the National Care Hotline was launched by the Ministry for Social and Family Development [MSF] in April 2020) set up during COVID-19.

## Conclusion

Telecommuting has been a boon to many and a bane to some, and this chapter has focused on two groups of WFH employees who may face the most challenges: parents with young children and the elderly. As companies and individuals settle into their WFH arrangements, a glimpse into the horizon might see telecommuting, in varying degrees, to remain or be adopted in some industries (Guyot & Sawhill, 2020; O'Mara, 2020). Whether it is the next pandemic that propels the next period of mandatory stay-home measures, it is hoped that these five psychological tips would serve as a meaningful guide for employees to be equally successful at home and in the workforce.

## Acknowledgement

The views expressed in this chapter are the authors' only and do not represent the official position or view of the Ministry of Home Affairs, Singapore.

## References

Arbaje, A. (2020). Coronavirus and COVID-19: Caregiving for the elderly. *John Hopkins Medicine.* https://www.hopkinsmedicine.org/health/conditions-and-diseases/coronavirus/coronavirus-caregiving-for-the-elderly

Ashforth, B. E., Kreiner, G. E., & Fugate, M. (2000). All in a day's work: Boundaries and micro role transitions. *The Academy of Management Review, 25*(3), 472–491. https://doi.org/10.5465/AMR.2000.3363315

Bowcott, O. (2020, May 1). Labour: Livestream court cases during and after Covid-19 crisis. *The Guardian.* https://www.theguardian.com/law/2020/may/01/labour-livestream-court-cases-during-and-after-covid-19-crisis-justice

Centers for Disease Control and Prevention. (2020a, July 1). *Coping with Stress.* https://www.cdc.gov/coronavirus/2019-ncov/daily-life-coping/managing-stress-anxiety.html

Centers for Disease Control and Prevention. (2020b, May 20). *Talking with children about Coronavirus Disease 2019.* https://www.cdc.gov/coronavirus/2019-ncov/daily-life-coping/talking-with children.html?CDC_AA_refVal=https%3A%2F%2Fwww.cdc.gov%2Fcoronavirus%2F2019-ncov%2Fcommunity%2Fschools-childcare%2Ftalking-with-children.html

Cirillo, F. (2006). *The Pomodoro Technique.* http://www.baomee.info/pdf/technique/1.pdf

Collingwood, J. (2018, October 8). *The power of music to reduce stress.* Psych Central. https://psychcentral.com/lib/the-power-of-music-to-reduce-stress/

Craft, L. L., & Perna, F. M. (2004). The benefits of exercise for the clinically depressed. *The Primary Care Companion to the Journal of Clinical Psychiatry, 6*(3), 104–111. https://doi.org/10.4088/pcc.v06n0301

Ehmke, R. (2020). *Talking to kids about the Coronavirus.* Child Mind Institute. https://childmind.org/article/talking-to-kids-about-the-coronavirus/

Elsesser, K. (2020, April 13). Telecommuting parents seek out virtual babysitting—here's how it works. *Forbes.* https://www.forbes.com/sites/kimelsesser/2020/04/13/telecommuting-parents-seek-out-virtual-babysitting-heres-how-it-works/#3880b06d6005

Foy, D. W., Drescher, K. D., & Watson, P. J. (2011). Religious and spiritual factors in resilience. In Southwick, S. M., Litz, B. T., Charney, D., & Friedman, M. J. (Eds.), *Resilience and Mental Health: Challenges Across the Lifespan,* 90–102. Cambridge University Press.

Giurge, L. M., & Bohns, V. K. (2020, April 3). 3 tips to avoid WFH burnout. *Harvard Business Review.* https://hbr.org/2020/04/3-tips-to-avoid-wfh-burnout.

Guyot, K., & Sawhill, I. V. (2020, April 6). Telecommuting will likely continue long after the pandemic. *Brookings.* https://www.brookings.edu/blog/up-front/2020/04/06/telecommuting-will-likely-continue-long-after-the-pandemic/

Heilweil, R. (2020, March 27) This social network for churches is thriving in the coronavirus pandemic. *Vox.* https://www.vox.com/recode/2020/3/27/21194239/coronavirus-churches-online-pray-com

Lau, A. L. D., Chi, I., Cummins, R. A., Lee, T. M. C., Chou, K., & Chung, L. W. M. (2008). The SARS (Severe Acute Respiratory Syndrome) pandemic in Hong Kong: Effects on the subjective wellbeing of elderly and younger people. *Aging and Mental Health, 12*(6), 746–760. https://doi.org/10.1080/13607860802380607

Li, C., & Lalani, F. (2020, April 29). *The COVID-19 pandemic has changed education forever. This is how.* World Economic Forum. https://www.weforum.org/agenda/2020/04/coronavirus-education-global-covid19-online-digital-learning/

Maxwell, W. (2003). The use of gallows humor and dark humor during crisis situation. *International Journal of Emergency Mental Health, 5*(2), 93–98. https://psycnet.apa.org/record/2003-06829-005

McCombs, B. (2010). *Developing responsible and autonomous learners: A key to motivating students*. American Psychological Association. https://www.apa.org/education/k12/learners

Moreno, M. A. (2016, October 21). Media use for 5- to 18-year-olds should reflect personalisation, balance. *AAP News*. https://www.aappublications.org/news/2016/10/21/MediaSchool102116

Murphy, M. (2020, April 23). Three warning signs that your remote employees are starting to crack under the stress of working from home. *Forbes*. https://www.forbes.com/sites/markmurphy/2020/04/23/three-warning-signs-that-your-remote-employees-are-starting-to-crack-under-the-stress-of-working-from-home/#7a23682a2237

National Association of School Psychologists. (2020, February 29). *Talking to children about COVID-19 (Coronavirus): A parent resource*. https://higherlogicdownload.s3.amazonaws.com/NASN/3870c72d-fff9-4ed7-833f-215de278d256/UploadedImages/PDFs/02292020_NASP_NASN_COVID-19_parent_handout.pdf

O'Donnell, L. (2020, March 31). Balancing work and elder care through the coronavirus crisis. *Harvard Business Review*. https://hbr.org/2020/03/balancing-work-and-elder-care-through-the-coronavirus-crisis

O'Mara, M. (2020, May 19). Twitter could end the office as we know it. *The New York Times*. https://www.nytimes.com/2020/05/19/opinion/twitter-work-from-home.html

Paddock, C. (2018, January 29). Just 30 minutes of light exercise each day can benefit health. *Medical News Today*, MediLexicon International. https://www.medicalnewstoday.com/articles/320760

Radesky, J. (2016, October 21). Policy addresses how to help parents manage young children's media use. *AAP News*. https://www.aappublications.org/news/2016/10/21/MediaYoung102116

Rosenbaum, E. (2020, April 9). What we've learned about how remote work is changing us. *CNBC*. https://www.cnbc.com/2020/04/09/heres-what-we-know-about-how-remote-work-changes-us.html

Salazar, C. (2001, September). Building boundaries and negotiating work at home. In *Proceedings of the 2001 International ACM SIGGROUP Conference on Supporting Group Work*, 162–170. https://doi.org/10.1145/500286.500311

Shin, K. M., Cho, S. M., Shin, Y. M., & Park, K. S. (2016). Effects of early childhood peer relationships on adolescent mental health: A 6- to 8-year follow-up study in South Korea. *Psychiatry Investigation, 13*(4), 383–388. https://doi.org/10.4306/pi.2016.13.4.383

Teo, D. (2020, April 15). A third of Singaporeans feel more productive working from home. *HRM Asia.* https://hrmasia.com/a-third-of-singaporeans-feel-more-productive-working-from-home/

Terrell, K. (2020, March 9). *4 tips on working from home during the coronavirus outbreak.* AARP. https://www.aarp.org/work/working-at-50-plus/info-2020/coronavirus-working-from-home-tips.html

Wahba, P. (2020, April 20). The retailers that are smartest about shopping tech will finish on top after the coronavirus. *Fortune.* https://fortune.com/2020/04/20/coronavirus-retail-industry-ecommerce-online-shopping-brick-and-mortar-covid-19/

Waite, P., Button, R., Dodd, H., & Creswell, C. (2020). *Supporting children and young people with worries about COVID-19* [PDF File]. Universities of Oxford and Reading. https://emergingminds.org.uk/wp-content/uploads/2020/03/COVID19_advice-for-parents-and-carers_20.3_.pdf

Wersebe, H., Lieb, R., Meyer, A. H., Hofer, P., & Gloster, A. T. (2018). The link between stress, well-being, and psychological flexibility during an acceptance and commitment therapy self-help intervention. *International Journal of Clinical and Health Psychology, 18*(1), 60–68. https://doi.org/10.1016/j.ijchp.2017.09.002

World Health Organization. (2020a, March 18). *Mental health and psychosocial considerations during the COVID-19 outbreak.* https://www.who.int/docs/default-source/coronaviruse/mental-health-considerations.pdf

World Health Organization. (2020b). *Coping with stress during the 2019-nCOV outbreak* [Infographic]. Who.int. https://www.who.int/docs/default-source/coronaviruse/coping-with-stress.pdf

Young, M. (2020, March 31). Working parents dealing with coronavirus quarantines will face psychological challenges. *The Conversation.* https://theconversation.com/working-parents-dealing-with-coronavirus-quarantines-will-face-psychological-challenges-134498

# Chapter 16

# Non-compliance with COVID-19 Safe Distancing Measures: Tips from Crisis Negotiators to De-escalate Situations

Xingyu Ken Chen, Nur Aisyah Abdul Rahman,
and Shannon Ng

## Introduction

Recently, there have been reports of safe distancing ambassadors (SDAs) being physically assaulted or verbally abused during their duties (Phua, 2020a; 2020b). Such incidents have raised concerns about the safety of officers who ensure that the community observe safe distancing guidelines such as wearing masks and following the one-metre rule when standing in queues. This chapter draws best practices from the field of investigative interviewing, crisis negotiation, and healthcare to inform the work of our SDAs. These practices are intended to complement the existing rules of engagement that officers have. These practices could potentially increase the success of engagement and de-escalate tense situations that they may encounter.

## Why Some People do not Comply

Since late-January 2020, there was a slew of measures introduced to combat community spread of COVID-19 with the emergence of the virus in Singapore. These include wearing of masks and a one-metre distancing between individuals in queues, among others. Additionally, SDAs from various government agencies have been appointed to help encourage the adoption of such measures in the community.

While most of the local community has adapted and adhered to such measures, a minority has been reported in the local news for non-compliance. An even smaller group have resorted to anti-social activities (e.g., bribery, verbal abuse, physical violence), which negatively impact the work that law enforcers and SDAs do to keep the community safe from COVID-19. Such non-compliance behaviours are inevitably a result of stressful changes brought on by COVID-19. Recent studies identified some common reasons people do not comply with these measures: loss of income, personal concerns about mental and physical health, and belief that they have done enough to protect themselves (Bodas & Peleg, 2020; Moore *et al.*, 2020). The fear of infection and job instability coupled with the sudden need to adapt to unfamiliar and inconvenient circuit breaker measures are stressors that can exacerbate existing life stressors and result in intense and difficult engagements with law enforcers and SDAs.

Another reason could be psychological reactance, which occurs when a person feels that someone or something is taking away their choices or limiting the range of alternatives (Steindl *et al.*, 2015). This feeling motivates them to restore their freedom by doing what they would normally do (e.g., not wearing masks), or complain about others who are flouting the same rules, or in some cases, act aggressively against the person telling them not to flout safe distancing practices. Psychological reactance towards requests to comply with safe distancing measures can also be a form of negative coping, as the person may do it to vent their negative emotions at the law enforcers and/or SDAs.

From the existing research and observing local cases, individuals who may be at a higher likelihood of non-compliance include those as mentioned in the following Table 16.1.

## Increasing Engagement Success

The key elements to persuading individuals to comply peacefully to the safe distancing measures are ultimately about rapport, and showing an understanding of the other party's concerns. The practices outlined here cover the entirety of an engagement process, ranging on how to approach

Table 16.1.   Individuals with higher likelihood of non-compliance.

| Potential groups | Possible reasons for non-compliance |
|---|---|
| General public | • Physical or mental health (e.g., "Staying at home all day is driving me crazy").<br>• Thinking that they are unlikely to contract the disease (e.g., "I am young, this disease only affects old people").<br>• Thinking that they are already well-protected from the disease (e.g., "I use hand sanitisers, I am well-protected already").<br>(see Dunning & Pownall, 2020; Moore *et al.*, 2020) |
| Elderly | • Misinformed about the disease.<br>• Think that threat is exaggerated.<br>• Preference for routine.<br>• Fearing the loss of agency and autonomy due to changes.<br>(see Petersen, 2020; Swant, 2020) |
| Non-locals | • Unfamiliar with local norms.<br>• Not updated with local COVID-19 measures and/or difficulty in adjusting. |
| Individuals with active mental health episodes* | May appear disoriented or confused, unable to focus and/or understand rules or instructions (Romo, 2018; Sabella, 2014).<br>*Common identifiers:*<br>■ Raised voice   ■ High-pitched voice   ■ Rapid speech<br>■ Pacing   ■ Fidgeting   ■ Excessive sweating<br>■ Excessive hand gestures   ■ Shaking   ■ Balled fists<br>■ Erratic movements   ■ Aggressive posture   ■ Verbally abusive<br>■ Hallucinations   ■ Poor personal hygiene   ■ Impacted speech: Made up words/goes off-topic |
| Individuals under the influence of alcohol or drugs | Unable to follow the rules or instructions due to intoxication ("How can I", 2019; "Tell-tale signs", 2016).<br>Some tell-tale physical signs are:<br>■ Blood-shot eyes   ■ Possession of alcohol/drugs   ■ Slurred speech<br>■ Excessive hand gestures   ■ Smell of alcohol   ■ High energy and confidence<br>■ Raised voice   ■ Loss of coordination   ■ Trembling/twitches<br>■ Paranoia   ■ Hallucinations   ■ Panic attacks<br>■ Sweating   ■ Slow response |

*Note:* *Not all with mental illness are violent and/or have active mental health episodes. Only a small minority with specific conditions may present with such symptoms. People living with mental health issues are not more prone to violence or non-compliance than the general population (Sabella, 2014).

a subject to de-escalate a tense situation. These practices are also applicable for cases when an officer encounters rising tension when they issue summons to a member of the public.

## *Part I: A Good Introduction*

Prior to engagement, officers can mentally prepare for the engagement by thinking through "what they want to say", and "how they want to say". A good introduction is critical to rapport-building as it helps to reduce the uncertainty of the engagement and prepares the subject for what to expect. Officers can engage people by first introducing themselves using the following steps as illustrated in Table 16.2.

Additionally, officers can build initial rapport with the subject by engaging in small talk with them. By engaging in small talk, it can help to create a relaxed atmosphere and produce positive feelings about the officer (Shaughnessy *et al.*, 2015). Some small talk examples include asking where the subject was from, the weather, the news, etc. (Pullin, 2010; Shaughnessy *et al.*, 2015).

Table 16.2.   How officers can introduce themselves.

| Steps | Example |
|---|---|
| 1. Maintain an appropriate physical distance. | Keeping a one-metre distance |
| 2. Personal Introduction. | "Hello, my name is …" |
| 3. Ask how would the subject like to be addressed. | "Sir/Madam, how may I address you?" |
| 4. Explain one's role. | "I am a safe distancing ambassador with the [Agency name]. Since COVID-19 my colleagues and I have been going around helping people adhere to safe measures such as xxx and xxx, so that together as a community, we can keep one another safe". |
| 5. Explain the purpose of the engagement. | "I notice you don't have your mask on, if not can I invite you to put own your own. Thank you", or "I've noticed you have not been observing the one metre safety distance in the queue… can I invite you to do that please?" |

## Part II: Active Listening of Concerns

Should the individual attempt to explain themselves, or protest against the request, an approach that officers could use to facilitate rapport would be to practice active listening. Active listening is not merely a passive act of listening, but showing the subject that the officer is paying attention, and is in tune with their explanations and emotions. Some of these active listening techniques recommended by crisis negotiators (Lanceley, 2003; Strentz, 2017; Voss & Raz, 2016) can be found in this section.

### Emotional Labelling

Emotion labelling is a skill to respond to the emotions heard in the subject's voice rather than the content. Emotion labelling usually starts with the words, "You sound/seem (emotion [e.g., angry] heard by the officer)". It is not telling a person how they are feeling (e.g., "You are upset"), but what they seem or sound like. Emotion labelling is useful as it gives a name to the feelings that the subject is experiencing, and shows that the officer is listening. However, emotion labelling is not appropriate in situations where the officer is verbally attacked. For example, if the subject is screaming at the officer, the officer should not say "You seem angry".

### Paraphrasing

Paraphrasing demonstrates that the officer is paying attention to what is being said. It is an act of summarising what the subject told the officer. Paraphrasing usually starts with the words "Are you telling me [what the officer heard]?)", or "Are you saying [what the officer heard]?". Paraphrasing is useful for a few reasons. It does not put the subject on the defensive, and it shows that the officer really understands and not merely parroting their concerns.

### Mirroring

Mirroring is repeating the last three words or crucial words as a question. For example, a subject might say, "I cannot exercise at all", and in turn, the officer can respond with "Cannot exercise at all?" to elicit more information about their frustrations. Mirroring can be useful in terms of asking for more information for the officer to act on. Even in instances where the officer is at a loss for words, it can help by encouraging the subject to keep talking.

## Silence

Silence is effective in getting the subject to talk. This is a simple act of staying silent, which can allow the subject to vent their emotions until they have calmed down. Silence can also be used to emphasise a point— the officer can use silence before they say something important, or after they have said something important.

## Minimal Encouragers

Minimal encouragers are words used to encourage the subject to continue talking by using simple phrases, such as "Yes", "OK", "Uh-huh", or "I see". This can effectively convey that the officer is now paying full attention to the subject, and all they have to say.

## Part III: De-escalating Tense Situations

Should an individual become agitated during the engagement, officers can consider adopting the use of de-escalation techniques to reduce the tension. Based on law enforcement and healthcare literature, this section provides four steps for de-escalating tense situations.

## Step 1: Set the Tone with Mutual Respect

Having one's sense of self or pride be vilified can be upsetting. In law enforcement literature, police officers' perceptions of disrespect and lack of cooperation by a subject, increase the likelihood of the use of force (Dayley, 2016). Treating the subject with dignity and minimising authoritativeness can help in tempering tensions (Todak, 2017). Zaiser and Staller (2015) found that perceiving and treating subjects as equals instead of aggravators, is crucial to setting the tone of the engagement with the subject. Effective de-escalators appear open, non-judgmental, confident, genuine, while not appearing arrogant (Price & Baker, 2012). There is a need to assert that you and the subject are partners in the community (e.g., "I know it can be a hassle, but you and I need to do our part for the community"). By doing this, it also empowers the subject to have a stake in the community's safety.

## Step 2: Control your Own Emotional Responses to Control the Situation

A situation can escalate quickly due to anger. Anger narrows the cognitive scope, which in turn, undermines one's cognitive control and rational thinking (Gable *et al.*, 2015). Non-compliant people might make physical attacks and/or verbally abuse the officer. Officers can retain control of the situation by avoiding angry emotional responses. They should remain calm and try to find out why the subject is refusing to comply. Communication occurs through body language, tone of voice, and word choice (Hallett & Dickens, 2015). Using a calm and professional tone of voice, and ensuring that what you say does not vilify or denounce the subject, can reduce aggravating the subject.

## Step 3: Listen and Find an Approach to get the Subject to Engage

Find ways to connect with the subject. Apply active listening skills to show empathy and build rapport. Some active listening techniques that can be used are covered earlier. Engaging the subject will allow officers to know more about them. For example, one can consider making small talk to find an approach to engage. Asking simple and non-threatening questions might also help to defuse some tension. This is a good way for officers to find leverage to persuade subjects to comply (e.g., "You mentioned that you have elderly parents. I can see that you are a caring son/daughter. COVID-19 is very dangerous for the elderly. I am sure that as a son, you want your parents to be healthy. Don't you think it best to do what you can to reduce any risk towards your parents?").

## Step 4: Provide Information and Support

Informing the subject that their actions can have legal ramifications can be effective for some people. However, there are those who are already aware that their actions are against the law and still refuse to comply.

These people might refuse to comply due to the feeling of loss in personal decision-making. Simply threatening the subject with the law and citing punishment, will only reinforce the feelings of personal disempowerment and further aggravate the subject. Hence, one can consider explaining the rationale behind social distancing measures (e.g., "There are people who might have the virus but do not appear sick. It is important everyone wears masks in public so that they do not get infected or spread the virus. Everyone has a role to play in keeping you and everyone else safe"). One can also reframe the situation and suggest alternatives (e.g., "How about exercising over there instead? There are fewer people there, so there is more space for you to move around"). Some subjects might be resistant and refuse to comply because they are misinformed about the COVID-19 situation. Thus, officers should attempt to clear up any misinformation that they might have, and guide them to reliable resources of information.

## *Ensure Personal Safety and Avoid Physical Engagement*

Ensuring personal safety and the safety of others is the number one priority. If the subject starts displaying threatening behaviour (e.g., increased voices, physical intimidation) and efforts to calm them down do not work, one should do the following: (1) do not physically touch/handle the subject, (2) disengage from the subject and move away from them, and (3) call 999 for help—get a colleague or member of the public to call the police, especially if the subject continues to engage you.

## Acknowledgement

The views expressed in this chapter are the authors' only and do not represent the official position or view of the Ministry of Home Affairs, Singapore.

## References

Bodas, M., & Peleg, K. (2020). Self-Isolation compliance in the COVID-19 era influenced by compensation: Findings from a recent survey in Israel. *Health Affairs*, 1–4. https://doi.org/10.1377/hlthaff.2020.00382

Dayley, E. H. (2016). Reducing the use of force: De-escalation training for police officers. [Master's Thesis]. Naval Postgraduate School. https://calhoun.nps.edu/handle/10945/50529

Dunning, A., & Pownall, M. (2020). Dispositional and situational attribution of COVID-19 risk: A content analysis of response typology, *PsyArXiv*, https://doi.org/10.31234/osf.io/czskd

Gable, P. A., Poole, B. D., & Harmon-Jones, E. (2015). Anger perceptually and conceptually narrows cognitive scope. *Journal of Personality and Social Psychology*, *109*(1), 163. https://doi.org/10.1037/a0039226

Hallett, N., & Dickens, G. L. (2015). De-escalation: A survey of clinical staff in a secure mental health inpatient service. *International Journal of Mental Health Nursing*, *24*(4), 324–333. https://doi: 10.1111/inm.12136

How can I tell if someone is using drugs? (2019, November 8). *Positive Choices.* https://positivechoices.org.au/parents/how-can-i-tell-if-someone-is-using-drugs

Lanceley, F. J. (2003). *On-scene guide for crisis negotiators* (2nd ed.). CRC press.

Moore, R. C., Lee, A., Hancock, J. T., Halley, M., & Linos, E. (2020). Experience with social distancing early in the COVID-19 pandemic in the United States: Implications for Public Health Messaging. *MedRxiv*, 1–4. https://doi.org/10.1101/2020.04.08.20057067

Petersen, A. H. (2020, March 12). How millennials are talking to their boomer relatives about the coronavirus. *Buzzfeed.* https://www.buzzfeednews.com/article/annehelenpetersen/coronavirus-parents-grandparents-boomers-millennials

Phua, R. (2020a, May 5). Woman filmed without mask, proclaiming "I'm a sovereign" to be remanded at IMH. *Channel News Asia.* https://www.channelnewsasia.com/news/singapore/sovereign-woman-shunfu-market-remanded-imh-12702696

Phua, R. (2020b, May 6). Man who stabbed NParks officer charged with attempted murder. *Channel News Asia.* https://www.channelnewsasia.com/news/singapore/covid-19-man-stabbed-nparks-officer-attempted-murder-12706090

Price, O., & Baker, J. (2012). Key components of de-escalation techniques: A thematic synthesis. *International Journal of Mental Health Nursing*, *21*(4), 310–319. https://doi:10.1111/j.1447-0349.2011.00793.x

Pullin, P. (2010). Small talk, rapport, and international communicative competence: Lessons to learn from BELF. *The Journal of Business Communication (1973)*. https://doi.org/10.1177/0021943610377307

Romo, J. (2018). The art of de-escalation and conflict resolution [PowerPoint slides]. http://www.napsa-now.org/wp-content/uploads/2012/06/De-escalating-Techniques-for-APS.pdf

Sabella, D. (2014). Mental illness and violence. *The American Journal of Nursing*, *114*(1), 49–53. https://doi:10.1097/01.NAJ.0000441797.87441.c9

Shaughnessy, B. A., Mislin, A. A., & Hentschel, T. (2015). Should he chitchat? The benefits of small talk for male versus female negotiators. *Basic and Applied Social Psychology*, *37*(2), 105–117. https://doi.org/10.1080/019735 33.2014.999074

Steindl, C., Jonas, E., Sittenthaler, S., Traut-Mattausch, E., & Greenberg, J. (2015). Understanding psychological reactance. *Zeitschrift Für Psychologie*, *223*(4), 205–214. https://doi.org/10.1027/2151-2604/a000222

Strentz, T. (2017). *Psychological aspects of crisis negotiation*. CRC Press.

Swant, M. (2020, March 13). HarrisPoll: U.S. seniors are least worried and least informed about COVID-19 but most at risk. *Forbes*. https://www.forbes.com/sites/martyswant/2020/03/13/harris-poll-us-seniors-are-least-worried-and-least-informed-about-covid-19-but-most-at-risk

Tell-tale signs of intoxication officers look for when making Minnesota DWI & DUI stops. (2016, November 30). *Judith Samson, Attorney at Law*. https://www.samson-law.com/signs-dwi-minnesota/

Todak, N. (2017). *De-escalation in police-citizen encounters: A mixed methods study of a misunderstood policing strategy* [PhD Thesis]. Arizona State University.

Voss, C., & Raz, T. (2016). *Never split the difference: Negotiating as if your life depended on it*. Random House.

Zaiser, B., & Staller, M. S. (2015). The word is sometimes mightier than the sword: Rethinking communication skills to enhance officer safety. *Journal of Law Enforcement*, *4*(5).

# Section 5

# Future Directions

# Chapter 17

# Surviving the Next Pandemic: Lessons for Humanity

Majeed Khader

## Introduction

As we began to write this book, it was clear that several issues were wanting. There were many useful lessons and some disappointments as we undertook this analysis. It is hoped that this concluding chapter captures the broad overarching issues which warrant some attention.

Beginning first with what we have to understand, some issues are clearer than others. In the chapters that followed earlier, they discussed the psychological and mental health impact of pandemics. Clearly, humans are affected. However, it does not seem naturally clear all the time that human sciences experts are needed in the solutioning. Across the world, it is not clear how governments have used psychologists, sociologists, and communication scientists to manage these crises. In fact, the psychological and mental health impacts appear to be an afterthought. Yet, for any one person who reports a fever (not necessarily COVID-19 related), many who hear about it begin to panic and become anxious. So clearly, there is a role for behavioural scientists and mental health professionals to play a part to assuage and manage the population, especially the "worried well".

Another important discussion within this book has been the chapters dedicated to the financial and economic impact of the COVID-19 crisis— jobs have been affected, some transformed, and many have ceased to exist. At face value, the solution seems deceptive; just help them get another job, or retrain them for other jobs. But, once again, as psychologists have long explained, a job is more than a month's wages; it is about life routine, psychological safety, sense of meaning, and dignity. In Asian societies, it is also about having "face". When one person is unemployed or has their business failing miserably, the entire family feels it.

From the broader community resilience angle, the role of the family in employment and unemployment, how religion may play a part in helping those during times of crises, embracing the new normal particularly in coping with the issues of telecommuting, bereavement, misinformation, and cyber wellness are all critical aspects to consider, and many of the chapters have discussed these.

From the angle of discussing those undertaking frontline jobs, some chapters within this book have discussed operational and organisational functioning considerations, and these are also as important, since if the frontline falters, the crisis of a pandemic would just worsen. In the Singapore context, when the circuit breaker was imposed, there were many questions about telecommuting, on-boarding, and non-compliance, and several chapters discussed these broader societal concerns.

Crises are often defined in terms of a lack of clarity which makes crisis handling, crisis management, and crisis leadership remarkably a difficult task. Rosenthal and Kouzmin (1977) referred to this as "unness", and the difficulty of defining clearly what exactly a crisis is and what the features of a crisis may be. Therefore, what were the realisations that behavioural scientists and practitioners have discovered? The following are some observations.

## *We Need More International "Meetings of Minds" to Better Appreciate the Psychological, Behavioural, and Sociological Impacts of the COVID-19 Crisis*

Firstly, while this crisis is biological in nature, it is apparent that the psycho-social footprint has been significant. Lives have been impacted in almost every country in the world. While it is acknowledged that there has been a psychological impact and a splattering of studies worldwide, it is also clear that these research pieces appear to be addressing different issues. There is no comprehensive understanding of the mental health impact of this COVID-19 crisis. There may be a need for world mental health experts to gather (perhaps virtually) to appreciate the global impact of the crisis on humanity. When we do not do so, our understanding of the psychological impact resembles the proverbial person holding onto different parts of the elephant, thinking that they understand the whole. There are many questions to be asked, but two primary ones ought to be: (1) how pandemics impact us psychologically, and (2) how do we manage this individually, in our communities, and globally? We need both local and global understanding. International collaborative studies, analyses, and discussions are needed. Experts have explained that this may not be the last crisis we will see, and we may see a resurgence of similar biological crises. Hence, we must identify and learn real lessons quickly. The learnings should not just be from the medico-biological front; it should equally be from the psycho-social sciences and humanities front.

## We Need to Understand the Precise Impact of the Pandemic Crisis on the Population at Large and for Specific Sectors and Respond Accordingly

Some of the questions that need answering are, what is the impact of the crisis on the population at large, and what is the sector-specific impact of the crisis? At the societal level, the question is defining if this is a generational crisis of the magnitude of other global crises, or perhaps not? The rates of casualty and property damage are, of course, markedly different. However, the similarities appear to be the shared human stress experiences that an entire generation goes through. This experience may not be entirely a negative one, but perhaps one that may energise populations and nations if they are positively appraised. National sense-making may turn bitter experiences to better experiences. Thus, the national collective healing efforts in managing the population psyche is critical. In this regard, the efforts by helping agencies have been a critical response. For example, in Singapore, we saw speedy responses from Silver Ribbon (Singapore), Fei Yue Community Services, Singapore Psychological Society, and also the provision of a National CARE Helpline (Ho *et al.*, 2020).

The second level of consideration should be focused on differential stress impact on specific groups of people. How did COVID-19 impact sectors differently, and which sectors are hard hit? For example, vulnerable groups such as low-income families, families with disabilities and mental illness, youth, and the elderly may experience a sense of vulnerability and loneliness with nationwide lockdowns and social distancing. The digital natives may not even experience digital connectedness with others. The lockdowns across the world have seen an increase in domestic violence and child abuse. Studies found an increase in gender-based violence, and this exacerbated preexisting gendered risks and vulnerabilities in Palestine, Mexico, and Brazil. In places like Chile and Bolivia, the decrease in help-seeking calls appears to suggest the inability of women to seek help through official channels (Bettinger-Lopez & Bro, 2020). In Singapore, the police reported a 22% rise in offences related to domestic violence, and from 7 April to 6 May 2020, there were 476 police reports. We have realised through this experience that not every house is a home for some, and more support needs to be provided. If the pandemic only lifted the lid on this harsh reality of home-related tensions, perhaps more professional studies are required to ease the nature of strained relationships at home?

## We Should Become Better at the Science and Art of Crisis Leadership

Did we learn from past crises? If we did, why are we not preventing the next pandemic when we have been thinking and planning to manage pandemics for a long time? Logically, given our collective experience in managing previous crises such as the Ebola, H1NI, Avian Flu, and Middle East Flu, among others, humanity ought to have been better able to handle the COVID-19 crisis. Why did we struggle to contain this? What "signal detectors" and sensing mechanisms have failed? Is there a playbook for good crisis handling? Clearly, these are some areas worth exploring:

a. Do we need better training for crisis leaders, including political leaders, government leaders, and medical crisis managers? We are of the view that the Singaporean experience has had some challenges. However, given the metropolitan type settings in Singapore where people are living in close proximity, the COVID-19 crisis is broadly speaking, very well managed. Strong political leadership, government transparency, strong communications, constant and almost daily updates, and a good relationship between the government and its citizenry may have helped in Singapore's case. However, not all countries have the same experience. History has shown that some leaders naturally emerged and shined during crises. Rudy Giuliani and

Winston Churchill are some examples. Lee Kuan Yew and his partnering co-leaders, who emerged from post-separation Singapore, were shining examples of crisis leaders who worked well as a team, were superb crisis communicators and excellent sense makers.

b. If we were to expect future pandemics, should medical and allied professionals like lab technicians, psychologists, social workers, require training in crisis leadership and crisis management? If they are a part of the machinery in crisis handling and advising political and government leadership, then this may be important. Future crisis will need to see a role for experts and professionals such as cyber and technical experts, biological experts, and psych-social experts—while they will not be leading the response to the crises, they are valuable allies to crisis leaders.

## *We Need Better Resilience in our Organisational and Human Systems*

In an efficient world, there seems to be no or little room for redundancy. Every system is tightly coupled with each other. Economies are closely linked and depend on each other, family routines are interlinked to work, work is interlinked to school, school vacations are interlinked to work schedules, tourism, and organisational output. However, when a crisis hits, this results in a domino effect where one system failure impacts another and yet another. Crisis experts have referred to this as a "snowballing effect". In fact, these effects were noted in several crises such as the 9/11 attacks and the Asian Tsunami. Despite these, modern living tends to lean towards complete interdependencies for the sake of being efficient. However, as crises impact us, these efficiencies fail, and there is no re-boot or failsafe solutions. It is clear, therefore, that solutions are needed in at least two areas.

The first is in systems design. When we design our economies and societies, it may be critical to consider that we do not become victims of a "domino" or "snowballing" effect, resulting from a crisis. This is referred to as "coupling", where one part of a system can influence other parts of complex systems (Strogatz, 2014).[1] Part of the discipline of

---

[1] Professor Steven Strogatz explains that "increasing the coupling between the parts seems harmless enough at first. But then, abruptly, when the coupling crosses a critical value,

thinking in this manner is to think about what the critical inter-dependencies can be, where they are situated, and how much redundancy we may need to have if one system fails. For example, if a nation's food security is impacted, are there contingency solutions? If the power supply is cut, what buffers might there be? Can internet disruption cause death and confusion in hospitals? Professor Randolph Nesse, Professor of Psychiatry and Psychology at the University of Michigan, explained that if complex systems (which are interconnected) fail, then "social chaos is just a pallid phrase for the likely scenarios [of panic]" (Nesse, 2014).

Given all of this, what is needed? What is needed is a deep appreciation of the hidden fragilities of complex systems we have in our countries. The danger is that sometimes we miss the "forest for the trees". By this, risk analysts may focus on the superficial threats of this or that, rather than the inherent design vulnerabilities (and design resilience) of our complex interconnected systems. Taking the COVID-19 crisis as an example, the issue may not be just about finding the right vaccine, but figuring out why the pandemic occurred in the first place. Was it the consumption of wild animals, or the human encroachment on nature? Medical experts explain that the virus is the third zoonotic coronavirus, after SARS-CoV and MERS-CoV (Mackenzie & Smith, 2020). So, as much as we want to rush to find the next vaccine, we do want to appreciate the deeper issues surrounding the roots of the problem. Hopefully, we become better learners and mitigate the next crisis.

The second issue pertains to human systems such as societies, families, and individual resilience. One reason why different people in different nations manage their crises differently (some better than others) is because some societies face crises often enough that their communities are mentally ready and remain resilient. They have a "crisis-ready mindset". How do we build this mindset? Some commentators have said that this crisis-ready mindset is found more in rural than in urban areas, since urban dwellers often rely heavily on government during times of crises. The question then is how we enable and empower our citizens to be self-sufficient and self-reliant to weather not just future pandemics, but also other kinds of "pan-global" crises? What would these "other" pan-global crises be? Whatever they might be, it is clear we need to train our

---

everything changes. The exact nature of the altered state isn't easy to foretell. It depends on the system's details. But it always something qualitatively different from what came before. Sometimes desirable, sometimes deadly".

policymakers, political leaders, crisis leaders, allied professionals involved in crisis management, and most importantly, our communities. We may need more training and exercises within our communities that mentally prepare us for these kinds of social and community crises.

## Acknowledgement

The views expressed in this chapter are the author's only and do not represent the official position or view of the Ministry of Home Affairs, Singapore.

## References

Bettinger-Lopez, C., & Bro, A. (2020). A double pandemic: Domestic violence in the age of COVID-19. *Council on Foreign Relations*. https://www.cfr.org/in-brief/double-pandemic-domestic-violence-age-covid-19

Ho, C. S., Chee, C., & Ho, R. (2020). Mental health strategies to combat the psychological impact of coronavirus disease 2019 (COVID-19) beyond paranoia and panic. *Ann Acad Med Singapore, 49*(3), 1–6. http://www.annals.edu.sg/pdf/49VolNo3Mar2020/V49N3p155.pdf

Mackenzie, J. S., & Smith, D. W. (2020). COVID-19: a novel zoonotic disease caused by a coronavirus from China: what we know and what we don't. *Microbiology Australia, 41*(1), 45–50. https://doi.org/10.1071/MA20013

Nesse, R. (2014). The fragility of complex systems. In J. Brockman (Ed), *What should we be worried about?: Real scenarios that keep scientists up at night.* Harper Collins.

Rosenthal, U., & Kouzmin, A. (1997). Crises and crisis management: Toward comprehensive government decision making. *Journal of Public Administration Research and Theory, 7*(2), 277–304. https://doi.org/10.1093/oxfordjournals.jpart.a024349

Strogatz, S. (2014). Too much coupling. In J. Brockman (Ed), *What should we be worried about?: Real scenarios that keep scientists up at night.* Harper Collins.